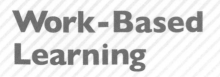

Work-Based Learning

Level 2

AWARD
CERTIFICATE
& DIPLOMA

DEMENTIA

Yvonne Nolan

ALWAYS LEARNING

PEARSON

Published by Pearson Education Limited, Edinburgh Gate, Harlow, Essex, CM20 2JE.

www.pearsonschoolsandfecolleges.co.uk

Heinemann is a registered trademark of Pearson Education Limited

Text © Yvonne Nolan 2012
Typeset by Tek-Art, Crawley Down, West Sussex
Original illustrations © Pearson Education 2012
Illustrated by Tek-Art, Crawley Down, West Sussex
Cover design by Pearson Education 2012
Picture research by Emma Whyte
Cover photo/illustration © Getty Images: Blend images/Jasper Cole

First published 2012

16 15 14 13 12
10 9 8 7 6 5 4 3 2 1

British Library Cataloguing in Publication Data

A catalogue record for this book is available from the British Library

ISBN 978 0 435 07788 4

Printed in Spain by Grafos S.A.

Every effort has been made to contact copyright holders of material reproduced in this book. Any omissions will be rectified in subsequent printings if notice is given to the publishers.

Pearson Education Limited is not responsible for the content of any external Internet sites. It is essential for tutors to preview each website before using it in class so as to ensure that the URL is still accurate, relevant and appropriate. We suggest that tutors bookmark useful websites and consider enabling students to access them through the school/college intranet.

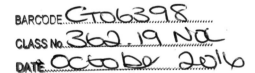

Contents

Acknowledgements iv

How to use this book v

Special features vi

1 Dementia awareness **1**
(DEM 201)

2 Person-centred approach to the care and support of individuals with dementia **27**
(DEM 202; DEM 204)

3 Communication and interaction with individuals who have dementia **49**
(DEM 205; DEM 210)

4 Equality, diversity and inclusion in dementia care **77**
(DEM 207; DEM 209)

5 Approaches to enable rights and choices for individuals with dementia whilst minimising risks **101**
(DEM 211)

Glossary 129

Further reading and research 131

Table of unit numbers by awarding organisation 133

Index 134

Acknowledgements

The publisher would like to thank the following for their kind permission to reproduce their photographs:

(Key: b-bottom; c-centre; l-left; r-right; t-top)

Alamy Images: 67photo 63, ACE STOCK LIMITED 8, Corbis Bridge 43b, 98, 119, Catchlight Visual Services 37, Corbis Bridge 43b, 98, 119, Fancy 47, Corbis Flirt 24, Richard Green 41, i love images / seniors 9, Image Source 107, Juice Images 87, Moodboard 29, 31, Moodboard 29, 31, PhotoAlto sas 55, Photofusion Picture Library 14r, Radius Images 91, Chris Rout 23tc, Science Photo Library 112, David Taylor 121, vario images GmbH & Co.KG 92; **Corbis:** Robin Bartholick 22, Najlah Feanny 82; **Fotolia.com:** Dan 27, Hr 49, Kostyantyn Ivanyshen 101; **Getty Images:** Bruce Ayres 94, Compassionate Eye Foundation / Jetta Productions 53, Comstock 10, ERproductions Ltd 20, Macduff Everton 2, Matthieu Spohn 116, Symphonie 34, Tetra Images 39; **Pearson Education Ltd:** Gareth Boden 32; **Pearson Education Ltd:** Image Source 23tr, 97, Lord & Leverett 96bl, Jules Selmes 33; **Shutterstock. com:** AJP 96br, andras_csontos 64b, Anette Linnea Rasmussen 1, Yuri Arcurs 95, Arpi 44, auremar 72, Matthew Benoit 64t, Blend Images 60, Joggie Botma 119b, Jim David 61, Durden Images 43, fotoluminate 80, Kardash 77, wong yu liang 96t, mangostock 23tl, Monkey Business Images 23cr, Galushko Sergey 114; **St Lawrence's Lodge:** St Lawrence's Lodge 120; **talkingmats.com:** 74

Cover images: *Front:* **Getty Images:** Blend images / Jasper Cole

All other images © Pearson Education

We are grateful to the following for permission to reproduce copyright material:

Table on page 20 of prevalence rates of dementia across the UK. Used with permission from the Alzheimer's Society www.alzheimers.org.uk; Text on page 42 of the ten commandments framework for approaching someone with dementia, adapted from the website of Alzheimer Belgium www.alzheimer.be. Used with permission from Alzheimer Europe www.alzheimer-europe.org; Text on pages 72–3 of suggestions for supporting communication with people who have dementia. Used with permission from Christine Bryden (www.christinebryden.com), author of *Who will I be when I Die?* and *Dancing with Dementia* (Jessica Kingsley Publishers, London).

Every effort has been made to trace the copyright holders and we apologise in advance for any unintentional omissions. We would be pleased to insert the appropriate acknowledgement in any subsequent edition of this publication.

How to use this book

Welcome to the Level 2 book to accompany the Dementia units for health and social care. The content of this book is intended to meet your needs if you are studying for the Award in Dementia Awareness, the Certificate in Dementia Care or the Dementia pathway of the Diploma in Health and Social Care.

This book covers five topics:

1 dementia awareness

2 taking a person-centred approach

3 communication

4 equality, diversity and inclusion

5 enabling rights and choices.

Three of these topics cover both a knowledge unit and a competence unit. This is because the content of the units is usually identical. In the margins of these chapters, you will see that it clearly signposts which criteria are covered in each section. To make it easy to track, the knowledge unit references are in red and the competence unit references are in blue.

For example:
AC 205:1.3 and 210:1.1

This section covers assessment criteria 1.3 from the knowledge unit and 1.1 from the competence unit.

You may find that you do not need to look at these references, but you can be sure that all the assessment criteria for the topics are covered in this book.

Special features

Look out for the following special features as you work through the book.

Case study

Real-life scenarios that explore key issues and broaden your understanding

Activity

A pencil and paper icon marks opportunities for you to consolidate and/or extend learning, allowing you to apply the theoretical knowledge that you have learned in health and social care situations

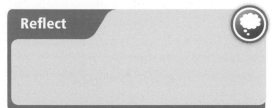

Doing it well

Information around the skills needed to perform practical aspects of the job. These are often in the form of checklists that you can tick off point by point to confirm that you are doing things correctly

Reflect

Reflect features have thought bubbles, to remind you that they are opportunities for you to reflect on your practice

Key term

Look out for the keyhole symbol that highlights these key terms – clear definitions of words and phrases you need to know

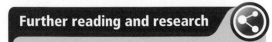

Getting ready for assessment

Information to help you prepare for assessment, linked to the learning outcomes for the unit

Further reading and research

Useful for continuing professional development, including references to websites, books and agencies

Chapter 1: Dementia awareness

This chapter is about developing your awareness of dementia: what it is and how it affects people. It is easy to think that everyone who has dementia is old and that nothing can be done about it. Neither of these ideas are true. Age is not the only factor that influences dementia, and there are many ways of reducing the effects of dementia and supporting people to manage the experience in a positive way.

This chapter provides an introduction and will touch on some areas that are covered in more detail in later chapters.

When you have achieved this unit you will:

- understand what dementia is
- understand the key features of the theoretical models of dementia
- know the most common types of dementia and their causes
- understand factors relating to an individual's experience of dementia.

1: Understanding dementia

1.1 What does the term 'dementia' mean?

Dementia is a term used to describe a disability caused by diseases or conditions that affect the brain and that causes problems with the way the brain functions. There are over 100 different conditions that can cause the symptoms of dementia. It is **not** a normal part of the ageing process.

Dementia is widespread: over 750,000 people in the UK are affected by dementia. The important thing to remember is that, while you need to understand the physical causes of the symptoms, people do not stop being people because they have dementia. Learning about how people's brains are affected by conditions and diseases is a vital part of understanding dementia, but dementia is not just a collection of symptoms to be dealt with.

The word 'dementia' is linked to the word 'demented' and so conjures up images of people being 'mad' or very disturbed, aggressive or dangerous. As a result, there is a fear of dementia and certain expectations of how people will behave. Most people have very little understanding of what dementia is like and what life is like for people who have it.

Dementia is a disability like any other. Your role is to support people and their families to live with their disability and get the very best out of life that they possibly can. In later chapters we will look in more detail at how to put people at the centre of everything you do.

Dementia is usually progressive. This means that symptoms will gradually increase as the brain becomes more damaged, and so the disability may become harder to live with. The speed at which the symptoms progress will vary, depending on:

- the circumstances of the individual (their physical and social environment)
- the individual's overall state of health and well-being
- medication, and the nature of the disease or condition that is causing the dementia.

People's abilities are likely to change over time.

Symptoms of dementia

The common **symptoms** of dementia are:

- memory loss
- communication difficulties
- changes in behaviour or mood.

We will look at each of these in turn.

Memory loss

People may find it hard to remember things that have just happened, or find it hard to understand what is happening in a television programme or a film. Sometimes even familiar routines such as going to the shops or making a meal may become confusing and hard to remember. The memory lapses will not be continuous, but people may notice that they become more frequent.

Key term

Dementia – a disability caused by diseases or conditions that affect the brain and that causes problems with the way the brain functions.

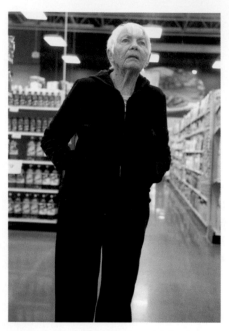

How do you think it would feel to forget familiar routines while you are out?

Key term

Symptoms – physical or mental indicators of a disease or injury.

Communication difficulties

Communication may sometimes be a challenge as people struggle to find the right word for everyday objects, or people's names. Others may struggle to recognise written words, or to make sense of what people are saying.

Communication difficulties can be made worse by age-related communication issues such as poor sight and hearing.

Changes in behaviour or mood

People with dementia may have sudden changes in behaviour and mood swings, behaving very differently than they have previously. They may express anger or frustration, or appear very low and depressed, or they may seem frightened and confused.

These changes in mood may be due to differing realities and difficulty in being able to understand the world around them. Moods can change quickly and everything may appear fine for a while. However, behaviour change is not only about changes to the brain. All behaviour is a means of communication, so the person with dementia may be using behaviour to express how they feel. It is important always to be aware of this and to think about what behaviour may mean.

Dementia is not a diagnosis in itself: it is the description of the disability that **results** from damage to the brain caused by a particular disease or condition. You will often hear the term used as if it is a condition or disease, for example, 'My mother's been diagnosed with dementia', or 'He used to be a lovely man, but he doesn't know anyone now because he's got dementia'. Dementia is a convenient way of describing the disability, but it is important that you remember that there is much more to dementia than one word.

> **Activity**
>
> Imagine you are writing a poster for a local senior citizens' organisation. You have been asked to give a brief explanation of dementia in no more than 50 words. What will you write?

1.2 How does dementia affect the brain?

The brain is the most complex organ in the human body: it is the 'control centre' for everything we do. Considering that it only weighs about 1.5 kilos, its activity is amazing. Our brain controls movement, speech, memory and behaviour. It keeps our bodies working and controls how we experience the world through our senses.

The brain is made up of billions of nerve cells. They are cells with long tentacles, a bit like an octopus. The tentacles connect cells to each other and pass messages through chemicals and minute electrical currents. If disease or injury breaks the connections between cells, they will die and the functions they performed will stop. Some cells in our bodies can regrow if they are injured: think about how skin heals when it has been cut. The nerve cells in our brain cannot do that. They simply die and stop functioning.

The brain is divided into four main sections:

- cerebral hemispheres
- limbic system
- cerebellum
- brain stem.

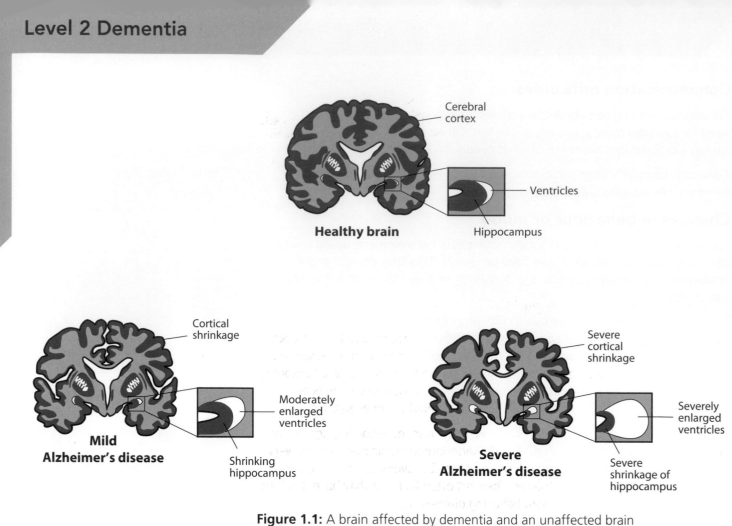

Figure 1.1: A brain affected by dementia and an unaffected brain

Each part of the brain has a specific task, as shown in Table 1.1 below.

Table 1.1: Functions of the four main sections of the brain

Area of the brain	Function
Cerebral hemispheres	'Grey matter' – divided into four lobes: each lobe performs a different job
Limbic system	Centre of the brain: responsible for learning and memory
Cerebellum	Controls balance, movement and posture
Brain stem	Controls body functions such as breathing, blood pressure and heartbeat

Cerebral hemispheres

The **cerebral hemispheres** make up most of the brain. They are the key areas that are affected by the conditions and diseases that result in dementia. When you hear the expression 'grey matter', this is what it means.

The cerebral hemispheres are divided into four lobes:

- frontal lobe
- temporal lobe
- parietal lobe
- occipital lobe.

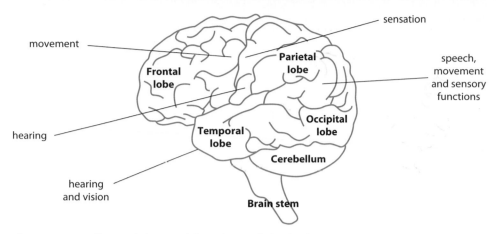

Figure 1.2: Different lobes and functions of the brain

The frontal lobe controls our behaviour. So when a disease or condition attacks the cells in this part of the brain, there are changes in people's usual behaviour. Someone who may have been very quiet can become loud and noisy, or outgoing and friendly people may become withdrawn and shy. A person who was always relaxed and laid back may become anxious and worried about everything.

This change in people's usual behaviour can result in them becoming aggressive or starting to lose their inhibitions, so their behaviour in public may become very challenging. Damage to the frontal lobe can cause behaviour changes that are very distressing for family and friends. They will often feel that they have 'lost' the person they knew as they see them behaving differently.

The temporal lobe provides important functions for language, emotion and memory.

Damage to the temporal lobe can mean that people have communication difficulties and may be unable to remember or recognise the words or sounds for everyday objects, or have difficulty joining in a conversation.

People may be unable to control their emotions: they may become very angry or very sad for no obvious reason. Sudden unexplained emotional changes can be hard to deal with for the person experiencing them – and for those around them.

The parietal lobe manages complex activities like detailed movements, and tasks such as calculating and spelling. Any damage to this area means that people may begin to lose the skills they once had in being able to work out finances, or to write letters.

The occipital lobe controls vision, so injury or disease in this lobe will affect sight. There are plenty of other age-related, and other, conditions that affect sight, so by no means are all vision impairments related to problems with brain functions.

Doing it well

At work, people with dementia will display all kinds of different behaviour. Some will be frightened, some will be happy and some will scream and shout.

Behaviour is about communication, so you need to think about what someone is trying to say to you. Don't just think about the physical things, like wanting a drink, being hot or cold, or wanting to go to the toilet. Think also about the emotional things, like wanting some company or some physical contact.

1.3 What other conditions can be mistaken for dementia?

> **Key term**
>
> **Depression** – severe dejection, accompanied by feelings of hopelessness and being inadequate.

Depression

The condition that is often mistaken for dementia is **depression**. People with depression can often experience memory loss, confusion, the inability to concentrate and the behaviour changes that are seen with dementia. In an older person it is particularly easy to mistake depression for dementia.

The treatments for the two conditions are very different and the prospects of recovery are also very different, so it is really important that a correct diagnosis is made. With the right treatment and support, people can make a good recovery from depression. Dementia is almost always progressive and can be slowed down, but not cured.

Stress

> **Key term**
>
> **Stress** – being under physical, mental or emotional pressure.

Stress can also cause confusion, lack of concentration and forgetfulness. People who are worried or overloaded with work and other demands on their time may find that they have a poor memory and feel confused or unsure sometimes. Stress can also cause mood swings and make people behave differently than they would usually. Often, as people get older, they assume that forgetfulness or lack of concentration is due to the ageing process, but stress should always be considered as a potential cause.

One of the key differences between someone with dementia and someone who is stressed or depressed is the ability to remember. A person who is depressed or very stressed will remember when they are reminded of what has been forgotten. A person with dementia will not usually respond even when they are reminded of the name they have forgotten, or the word they were looking for. They may pretend that they have remembered, but they will be unable to recall the information shortly afterwards. People with dementia can also have depression, which can make the diagnosis of dementia difficult. It is not always easy to identify the dementia symptoms, as they are similar to those of depression. This can result in dementia being diagnosed quite late.

Delirium

> **Key term**
>
> **Delirium** – mental confusion and changing levels of consciousness.

Delirium is a condition that is fairly common among older people. It has similar symptoms to those shown in dementia: people are confused and unable to communicate clearly. They may ramble or repeat themselves, or may swing wildly between being aggressive and being frightened and confused. Their sleep is often disturbed and they may not be aware of their surroundings.

The causes of delirium can include:

- illness/disease
- infection
- inflammation
- dehydration
- constipation
- malnutrition
- side effects of medication
- urine retention
- pain.

Delirium is different from dementia because its symptoms will improve once the cause is treated.

The onset of worsening symptoms of delirium, coupled with physical indicators, may highlight that a person is suffering from dementia as well as delirium.

Late-life forgetfulness (Mild Cognitive Impairment)

One of the conditions frequently assumed to be dementia is Mild Cognitive Impairment (MCI). The condition is also sometimes called late-life forgetfulness, which reflects its symptoms clearly. Late-life forgetfulness is what happens to many of us as we grow older: we cannot remember where we left the car keys, we forget appointments, phone numbers and people's names, etc.

This condition is not the same as dementia because the underlying ability to function and get on with day-to-day living is not seriously affected. You may forget your car keys, but you do not forget how to get home from the shops. You may not remember the name of the film you saw last week, but you can remember how to get dressed.

Late-life forgetfulness is caused by a range of factors, such as:

- slower absorption of key nutrients such as vitamin B12
- declining levels of hormones such as oestrogen and testosterone
- reduced levels of blood flow and oxygen to the brain.

It can also be made more likely by:

- not keeping the brain active, which is like a muscle – 'use it or lose it'!
- lack of exercise, smoking or poor diet.

Some key differences between dementia and late-life forgetfulness are shown in Table 1.2.

Table 1.2: Key differences between the symptoms of late-life forgetfulness and dementia

Possible symptoms of late-life forgetfulness (or Mild Cognitive Impairment – MCI)	Possible symptoms of dementia
You forget things, but can live a normal life and carry on your usual activities.	Day-to-day life is affected – you have difficulty paying bills, cooking a meal, getting dressed, and you have problems doing very familiar things.
When reminded, you can remember what you have forgotten and when, and can tell people about it.	You cannot recall, or are unaware that you have forgotten, information.
You sometimes forget the right word and have it 'on the tip of your tongue', but you can hold a conversation.	You have difficulty holding a conversation and may repeat things or get them mixed up.
You have not lost the wisdom and common sense you gained from life experience. You can still make judgements and sensible decisions.	You may not be able to make logical judgements or decisions, and behaviour may sometimes be inappropriate.
You may have to think about how to get somewhere, but you do not get lost in places you know well.	You can get lost in familiar places, and cannot follow directions.

A series of studies run by memory clinics quoted by the Alzheimer's society identified that 10–15% of people with MCI go on to develop dementia each year.

Jim is 71 years old. He is a retired postman and lives with his wife Joan. Their family lives locally and their three grandchildren visit regularly.

Lately Jim has become worried about his memory: for example, last week he forgot to meet his friend in the pub as he had arranged, and only remembered when his friend texted him. He keeps on calling his older grandson by his son's name. The other day he forgot his youngest grandson's name entirely when he was talking to an old friend, and only remembered when Joan said it. He finds that he frequently walks into a room and cannot remember what he came in for.

Jim does some pottering in the garden and keeps the house up to scratch. He also does odd jobs for his family. He and Joan go shopping and sometimes have days out when the weather is nice. Apart from that, he keeps up to date with the news on television and enjoys watching property and DIY shows.

Jim and Joan have been discussing his memory lapses and think that these may be the early signs of dementia. They are thinking about going to the GP.

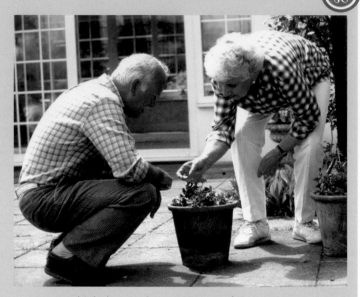

1 Do you think that Jim has symptoms of dementia?
2 Give two reasons why.
3 What may be the reasons for Jim's forgetfulness?
4 What do you think the GP will say to Jim and Joan?

2: Key features of the theoretical models of dementia

2.1 Medical model

Until the last few years, the medical model was the way in which all dementia was looked at and understood. The model works on the basis that dementia is incurable and is terminal. A great deal of research is being undertaken into the causes of dementia, its effects on the brain and ways in which it can be improved or its progression delayed. Individuals are assessed and the problems presented by their dementia are identified. Suitable services to meet their needs are discussed and agreed with people with dementia and their families.

There is a long history of medication use for people with dementia. People have been treated with anti-depressants, tranquillizers and anti-psychotic drugs, such as Aricept, in order to attempt to control the symptoms of dementia. The medical model is focused on how an individual's symptoms can be improved: the treatment will vary for each individual according to the severity of symptoms. Recently, government initiatives have aimed to reduce the use of anti-psychotic drugs because of the side effects and risks. Anti-psychotics have been described as the 'chemical cosh' – in other words, just a way of keeping people calm and quiet.

Managing the symptoms of dementia is the underlying basis of the medical model. Everything possible is done to ensure that people have symptoms under control and are as well as they can be. The model recognises the need for people to receive care and to have their needs met. This can be at home, or more often in a residential or nursing home.

Families and carers are supported to look after the person with dementia and are kept informed on all aspects of a person's care. Plans are developed in consultation with carers: risks to the person are considered and steps put in place to ensure that people are kept safe. For example, if a person wanders and gets lost, doors may have to be locked to prevent this from happening. If someone is becoming a serious risk at home then it may be inevitable that some form of residential care becomes necessary. Health professionals are usually key people providing support for individuals and families, along with social care professionals in both domiciliary and residential settings.

2.2 Social model

The approach of the social model is to see the whole person, not just a set of symptoms that need to be managed and treated.

People are who they are because of all kinds of factors and influences, including:

- their family
- their friends
- their education
- the job they have done
- their health and how well they are
- their accommodation
- their neighbours and local community.

In the social model, professionals take all aspects of a person's life into account when working with them to develop a support plan. This puts the person at the

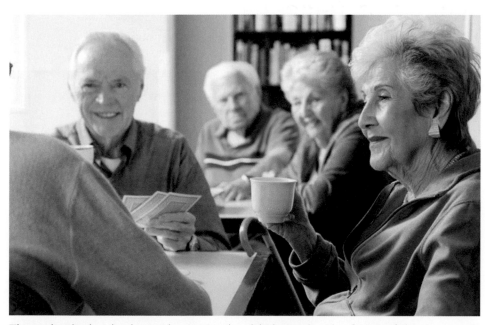

The individuals who have dementia should always be the focus of the support plan.

centre of everything. The job of the professionals is to support the process of someone deciding how they can make best use of the skills and abilities they currently have, and to plan for how these may change in the future.

Another key principle of the social model is to look at what people with dementia *can* do, and build on those areas, rather than focus on problematic factors. The model promotes the active involvement of people with dementia in all aspects of their support, and in all aspects of life as far as they wish.

This approach believes in the importance of maintaining the 'personhood' of people with dementia – in other words, not forgetting that they should be given the same respect and consideration as they were before they developed dementia. It is easy to forget that someone who now has very limited capacity has had the same kind of life experience as all of us. They have been a child, a teenager, perhaps had a career, been in love, got married, had children: all the usual phases and changes in a person's life. Just because some parts of their life story are fading from their memory does not mean that you can forget it too. People with dementia are still who they always were. People have likes and dislikes: they may be the same now as they have always been, or they may have changed, but they form part of that person's identity.

In later chapters we will look at the positive work that can be done to support people with dementia: to take maximum advantage of the capacity they do have, and to hold on to and improve their mental skills and abilities wherever possible. There may be things that a person can no longer do as well as they used to, but these can be overcome by choosing the right support package and by focusing on how routines and lifestyles can change in line with someone's changing abilities.

The environment in which people live is a key element of the social model. Environment is not only a person's immediate surroundings of home and family, but also their neighbours and local community.

Important environmental factors in supporting people to live with dementia include:

- the type of housing people live in
- the safety and accessibility of their local area
- the support available from community groups and neighbours.

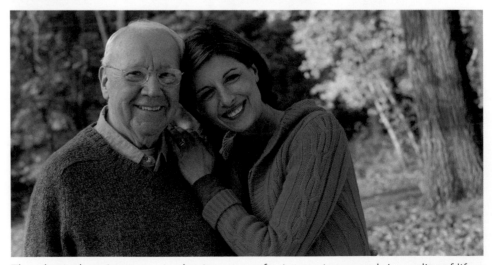

The physical environment is also important for improving people's quality of life.

The social model of dementia assumes that everyone can be fully understood: it just may take time and patience. Communication is a key aspect of understanding. Recognising that all behaviour is a means of communication is essential if people with dementia are to be understood.

2.3 Dementia is a disability

Dementia is a progressive, terminal disease, but it is important that it is also recognised as a disability.

The social model recognises that people can be disabled by the environment and the society in which they live. Here are a couple of examples:

- People who use wheelchairs to get around cannot use stairs. If a building has lifts and slopes instead of stairs and steps, then the ability of people using wheelchairs to access the building is no different from anyone else's.

- A person with profound deafness who watches a film with subtitles has a similar experience to someone who is not deaf, but if the film has no subtitles then they are excluded from that experience. It is not the deafness that disables the person watching the film – it is the fact that there are no subtitles.

The same principle applies to dementia. The circumstances in which a person with dementia lives and the way in which society and their local environment can adapt to meet their needs can make all the difference to how disabling the dementia is.

A good example of the areas that can make a difference is the 2007 World Health Organization publication, *The Global Guide to Age Friendly Cities*. The publication was the result of a survey undertaken in various cities around the world to see how easy it was for older people to live in them.

The areas that were looked at in the survey are shown in Figure 1.3.

Activity

Work out which model is used in your workplace by answering the following questions.

1　Is the model very clearly medical or clearly social?
2　Is the model a mix of the two?
3　How do you know?

Note down the main reasons you have for reaching your answer.

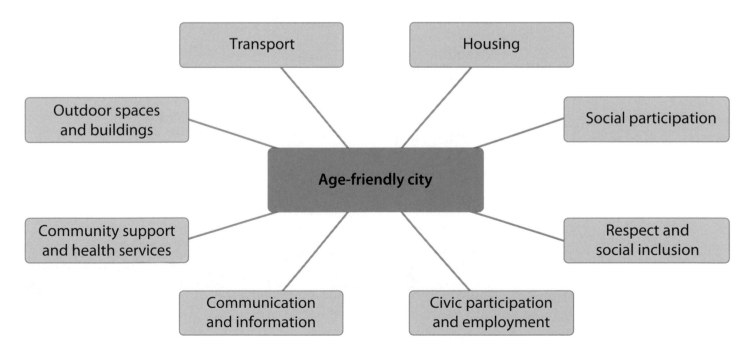

Figure 1.3: The environmental factors that can make a difference to how disabling dementia is

Activity

Think about your local town or city.

Consider the eight factors (or 'petals') in Figure 1.3. How well does your local area score for each of them?

All of these factors can help to create an environment that makes it easier for people to stay active, well and involved in local life. This can make a huge difference to how long people with dementia are able to maintain independence and remain in their own home.

A more positive approach to dementia can offer a better quality of life for people with dementia and their families, by looking at it as a disability to be lived with, rather than a disease to die from.

3: Know the most common types of dementia and their causes

3.1 The most common causes of dementia

The most common causes of dementia are:

- Alzheimer's disease
- vascular dementia
- Lewy body dementia
- fronto-temporal dementia.

Alzheimer's disease

Alzheimer's disease is the most common cause of dementia: it affects around 465,000 people in the UK each year. It is a progressive disease which means that over time, people become increasingly less able and need support in more areas of their lives.

The name of the disease comes from the German doctor who first described it: Alois Alzheimer. People with Alzheimer's develop certain proteins which cause 'tangles' to develop in the brain. There is also a loss of certain chemicals that appear to affect the transmission of messages in the brain.

Vascular dementia

Vascular dementia is the second most common cause of dementia after Alzheimer's disease. The term 'vascular' is used to refer to the blood vessels that carry blood around the body. The blood in the vascular system carries oxygen to all parts of the body, including the brain. In order for brain cells to work properly, they need a good supply of oxygen.

Certain conditions can cause damage to the vascular system, such as high blood pressure, diabetes, high cholesterol and heart disease. Strokes can also cause significant damage to the vascular system: either by having one major stroke, or sometimes many small strokes over a period of years.

Any of these conditions can reduce the amount of oxygenated blood circulating in the brain, and when this happens the brain cells gradually die. This results in the onset of vascular dementia.

Lewy body dementia

Lewy body dementia is similar in some ways to Alzheimer's disease. Lewy bodies (named after the doctor who identified them) are protein deposits that lodge in the brain and interrupt the sending of chemical messages in the brain.

Interestingly, Lewy bodies are also found on the brains of people with Parkinson's disease, but research has not yet identified why they occur or how the damage happens.

Fronto-temporal dementia

Have another look at Figures 1.1 and 1.2 from pages 4 and 5, which show diagrams of the brain.

Fronto-temporal dementia refers to any disease or condition that causes damage to the frontal or temporal areas of the brain. One of the most common causes of this type of dementia is Pick's disease, which causes proteins to be deposited inside cells in this part of the brain.

Research has not yet found out why this happens in certain parts of the brain more than others. Fronto-temporal dementia is not as frequent as some of the other causes of dementia, although it is far more common in people under the age of 65.

This is the only form of dementia where research has possibly identified a family link: some genes appear to be connected to this type of dementia. However, research is ongoing.

Other – rarer – conditions that can cause dementia include:

- HIV/AIDS
- Creutzfeldt-Jakob disease
- Korsakoff's syndrome.

HIV/AIDS

Sometimes people develop dementia symptoms in the late stages of HIV/AIDS.

Creutzfeldt-Jakob disease

Creutzfeldt-Jakob disease is rare in humans, but it has affected animals for many years. It is the result of an infection that attacks the nervous system and then gets into the brain.

Korsakoff's syndrome

Korsakoff's syndrome is named after the composer, Rimsky Korsakoff, who was said to have suffered from it. It causes short-term memory loss and is usually the result of serious alcohol abuse over many years.

Doing it well

Not everyone you work with will have the same cause for their dementia.

Make sure that you know the reason for a person's dementia. That way, you will be better able to understand the likely symptoms and know the best way to offer support. People can experience elements of more than one form of dementia. This is called 'mixed dementia'.

3.2 Signs and symptoms of dementia

Alzheimer's disease

Alzheimer's disease can only be confirmed by a proper diagnosis and medical tests.

However, the following symptoms may indicate Alzheimer's.

Short-term memory loss

People may be unable to remember events that have just happened, or they may repeat a question after just a few minutes. They may insist that they have to go shopping, even though they have just returned.

This type of memory loss also includes forgetting people – not just having difficulty with names, but forgetting who someone is entirely.

Misplacing or losing items

This happens to us all, but someone with Alzheimer's disease will be unable to recall where they have put something and, unlike most of us, will not even remember when it is found.

Another common symptom is that items may be found in strange places: a tin of beans in the bed, or a cardigan in the fridge. People can lose the ability to connect information about objects and where they should be.

Disorientation

People can become disorientated in terms of time and place.

The concept of time may no longer apply in their world – for instance, they may want to go shopping at 3am.

They can also become disorientated about where they are and not recognise familiar places, or they might frequently get lost and be unable to recall the way home. Sometimes people will become very distressed because they do not recognise their surroundings and have no idea where they are.

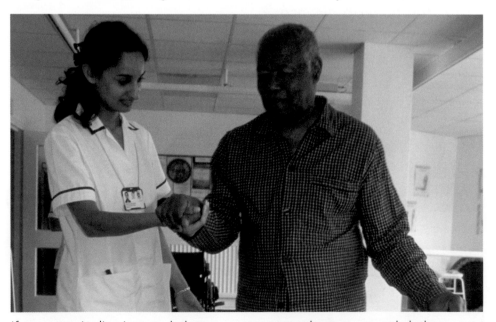

If someone is disorientated, the way you support them can greatly help to reduce their distress.

Communication challenges

Sometimes people may struggle to find the right words to hold a conversation, so they often use words that do not sound right in the context. There can often be a link to the word they are trying to remember, but it makes holding a conversation a challenge for them.

Struggles to communicate verbally often result in people trying to communicate through their behaviour. This can often be dismissed as agitation or aggression, adding to the frustration that the person with dementia is already experiencing.

Making judgements

People can become less able to make day-to-day judgements about risks and danger.

This can mean that people will go out in freezing temperatures in summer clothes or pyjamas, they will let strangers into their homes, or they are vulnerable to confidence tricksters and thieves. Sometimes people have been found walking on motorways, completely unaware of the danger.

Vascular dementia

Although the causes of vascular dementia are different to Alzheimer's disease, and the brain is affected differently, some of the symptoms are similar, such as memory loss, losing items and disorientation.

The symptoms of vascular dementia can vary, depending on which area of the brain has been affected, but they are likely to include the following.

Slower thinking process

People may become slower in the way they think, so that everything they do becomes slower and more difficult. It may take quite a while for someone to find the right word for a sentence, or they may lose track of what they were trying to think of and miss the word completely.

Mood swings

Mood changes and displays of emotions may become more frequent. People's behaviour can be very different to how they previously behaved: emotions can change from being tearful to being happy or being angry.

Mood changes are not always about brain changes. A lot of the changed behaviour in people with any type of dementia can be about frustration with their reducing capacity to do things, and also with the way that they are treated by professionals and society in general.

Mobility

For some people with vascular dementia, there may be a change in how they walk, or difficulty with walking and getting around. This may be one of the things that people notice early on.

If the dementia is following a stroke, then there may be mobility problems in any event.

Lewy body dementia

Lewy bodies has some symptoms in common with Alzheimer's disease and vascular dementia, such as memory loss and disorientation.

However, Lewy body dementia can show some quite distinct symptoms that are not necessarily found in other causes of dementia:

Visual hallucinations

Visual hallucinations can mean that people see things that are not real. However, they are very real to the person seeing them and can cause great distress and fear. It can often be very difficult to comfort and reassure someone who is hallucinating.

Vivid dreams

Along with hallucinations, people with Lewy bodies can also experience vivid dreams, and can move a lot when they are sleeping. Again, it is often hard to offer people comfort after very disturbing dreams.

Movement

People can experience some symptoms that may seem similar to Parkinson's disease, such as stiffness in the limbs, slow movement and a tremor. People may also have fainting episodes and be prone to falls.

Attention and alertness

People may show quite different levels of alertness and attention at different times. This can differ from hour to hour and can be very noticeable. Someone who was quite chatty and sharing a cup of coffee and a joke at 11am may not seem to know who you are by early afternoon, but be back to being alert and discussing the TV programmes in the evening.

Fronto-temporal dementia

Fronto-temporal dementia largely affects younger people between the ages of 30 and 60, although it can be sometimes found in older people.

The symptoms are different in many ways from other causes of dementia, although they sometimes look similar in the early stages, especially in communication issues such as forgetting words or people's names, or not understanding some words. Interestingly, in the early stages there is no memory loss, although it can seem as if there is because of communication problems.

Other symptoms can include the following.

Personality changes

People can appear to be rude or very impatient. They can also behave quite inappropriately in public, such as removing clothes or shouting loudly. Quite often there is a change in how someone reacts to other people: they may seem to lose any warmth or concern for others and behave in what seems like a selfish way.

Eating habits

It is quite common for people to crave sweet foods and to overeat, regardless of the sort of diet they may have followed in the past.

If this is coupled with personality changes, it can make life a challenge for the person concerned and for friends and family who are trying to understand what is happening.

3.3 Risk factors for dementia

Risk factors are those elements in someone's history or lifestyle that increase or decrease the chances of developing a particular condition.

There is a great deal of research being undertaken into dementia, so there is new information available regularly. The current view is that the risk of developing dementia is a combination of genetic and environmental factors.

The main factors are:

- age
- gender
- lifestyle
- family history/genetics.

We will look at each of these factors in turn.

Age

One in six people over 80 has dementia, as opposed to one in 100 between 65 and 70.

Age is the most significant factor and the one we can do least about. Although we all get older, this does not mean that we will all develop dementia, just that the risk is increased the older we get. There are younger people with dementia, and there are many older people who do not have it. One in five people over 80 do develop it, but four out of five do not.

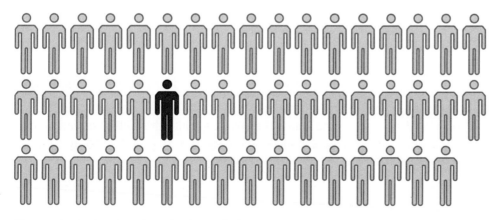

Figure 1.4a: One in a hundred people between 65 and 70 has dementia.

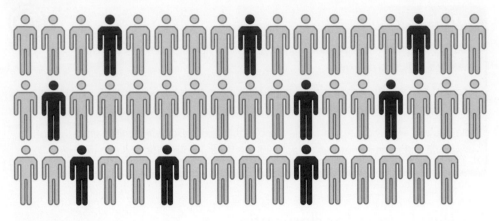

Figure 1.4b: One in six people over 80 has dementia.

Gender

Gender is another factor that we can do little to change.

Women are a little more likely than men to develop Alzheimer's disease, whereas men are slightly more likely to develop vascular dementia than women.

Lifestyle

Several of the factors that increase the risk of developing dementia are associated with the way we live.

Smoking, diet, exercise and alcohol consumption can all have an impact on the likelihood of developing dementia in older age.

Smoking

The effects of smoking on the lungs and vascular system are well known, as well as the risks of cancer and the increased risk of heart disease.

The health of brain cells depends on the brain's vascular system, so smoking is a significant risk factor for vascular dementia. Research has also shown that smokers are almost twice as likely as non-smokers to develop Alzheimer's disease.

Diet

The benefits of a healthy balanced diet are well known.

Maintaining a healthy body weight reduces the risk of developing conditions like high blood pressure or heart disease, both of which increase the risk of developing dementia.

The vitamins and antioxidants in fresh fruit and vegetables have been shown to prevent heart disease in some research studies. This reduces the risk of dementia.

Other studies indicate that polyunsaturated fatty acids, such as those in oily fish, may also have benefits for the heart. There is little doubt that saturated fats cause arteries to become narrowed and increase the risk of strokes and heart attacks, both of which are increased risk factors for dementia.

Exercise

There is strong evidence that maintaining physical activity throughout life protects against many diseases. In particular, exercise benefits the heart, lungs and vascular system, all of which are essential for keeping a healthy blood flow to the brain, reducing the risk of developing vascular dementia.

On the other hand, people whose form of exercise exposes them to head injury repeatedly or severely, such as boxers or some rugby players, are three or four times more likely to develop dementia.

Alcohol

Large amounts of alcohol over time increases the risk of developing Korsakoff's syndrome, a form of dementia specifically related to abuse of alcohol.

Recent research has shown that red wine in moderate amounts can help to keep the vascular system and brain healthy because of the antioxidants contained in it.

Family history/genetics

Research into the effect of genes on dementia is still ongoing: we learn something new regularly.

There has been progress in identifying some of the genes that relate to Alzheimer's disease. There is some evidence that a very small number of people may have a genetic link to some more unusual forms of Alzheimer's disease, where it starts before the age of 60. This is called 'early onset', as opposed to 'late onset' which is the most usual form of the disease.

There are some genetic conditions, such as Down's syndrome or Huntington's disease, that make it more likely that someone will develop Alzheimer's disease. Fronto-temporal lobe dementia appears to have a strong inherited link, and having a family member with the condition increases the risk of having it. People from black and minority ethnic communities have a higher chance of developing early onset dementia. There is more information about dementia in various communities in Chapter 4.

3.4 Prevalence rates for different types of dementia

Prevalence is the figure that shows *how often* something occurs, as opposed to **incidence**, which is always accompanied by a time frame (such as a year) and is about *how many* times something happens.

According to the Alzheimer's Society:

- in total there are about 750,000 people in the UK who have dementia
- over 16,000 of them are under 65.

Of the 750,000 people who have dementia:

- 62 per cent have Alzheimer's disease
- 17 per cent have vascular dementia
- 10 per cent have a mix of Alzheimer's and vascular dementia
- 4 per cent have Lewy body dementia
- 2 per cent have fronto-temporal lobe dementia
- 2 per cent have Parkinson's dementia
- 3 per cent have the rarer forms of dementia.

Prevalence rates across the UK are shown in Table 1.3.

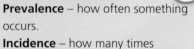

Key terms

Prevalence – how often something occurs.
Incidence – how many times something happens: always defined within a time frame (e.g. a year).

Table 1.3: Prevalence rates of dementia across the UK (source: Alzheimer's Society. Dementia UK, published 2007 (updated 2011)

Age	Prevalence
40–64	One person in every 1,400 of the population
65–69	One person in every 100
70–79	One person in every 25
80+	One person in every six

4: Understand factors relating to an individual's experience of dementia

4.1 Living with dementia

Having a **diagnosis** of dementia does not mean that someone should suddenly change their whole life and start living in a different way. There is no need to rush off into a hospital or residential care. For most people it is perfectly possible to remain at home and continue to live an independent life, with support that increases as necessary as the dementia progresses.

For many people a diagnosis can almost be a relief: it is confirmation that something is wrong. They may have suspected for a long time that all was not well, and they are finally able to know for sure what the problem is and get the help and support they need.

Living with dementia is not easy. Different types of dementia bring different problems. As you have learned earlier in the chapter, one type can bring mobility problems, another may result in frightening hallucinations. For everyone with dementia, there will be a gradual loss of memory and a loss of the ability to make sense of the world.

Key term

Diagnosis – identification of an illness by looking at the symptoms.

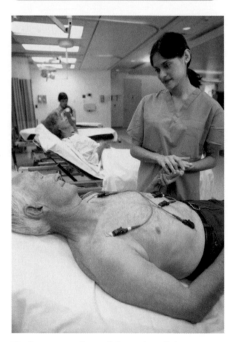

Before reading this unit, did dementia immediately make you think of old people in hospital?

Reflect

Try to imagine how frightening it would be if nothing made sense any more.

Think about an experience when you have been in a strange place, not sure of where you are or how to get back to where you want to be. You might have been visiting a different town, or perhaps in a maze.

Try to recall your feelings – maybe you were afraid, or perhaps just angry and frustrated. Think about how it might feel if that happened to you every day.

Have you ever been in a country where people speak a different language? How hard did you find it to communicate when nothing made sense? It might have all been part of the fun of a holiday, but how would it feel if that was constant, if much of what was being said to you did not make proper sense?

Although it is not easy, it is perfectly possible to live with dementia and to maintain independence and a fulfilled life for a considerable period of time after diagnosis.

Factors influencing how different people experience dementia

Many different factors influence how different people experience dementia. These are shown in Figure 1.5 and described in detail below.

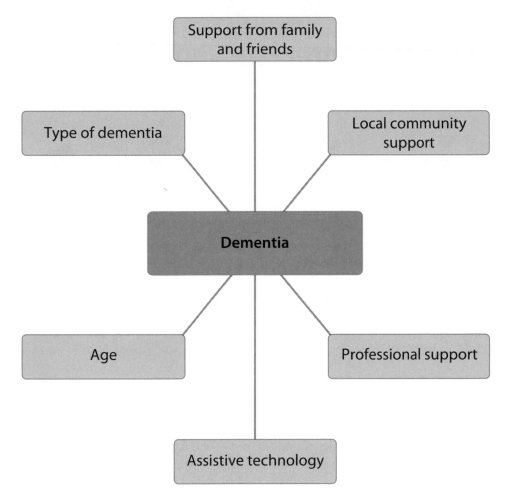

Figure 1.5: The factors that influence how different people experience dementia

Support from family and friends

For people with dementia, the ability to maintain control over choices about day-to-day living is important.

Having friends and family who are willing and able to be part of a support plan makes a huge difference to how long and how well people can maintain their lives as they wish.

Here are a few examples:

- Family and friends can do regular 'pop-in' visits to make sure that someone is OK.
- A family member or friend could be the contact point for alarms raised by assistive technology.
- A family member or friend could be the named person on a help card (see Figure 1.6).

I have an illness called dementia.

I would appreciate your help and understanding.

▼
▼
▼ ▶ ▶ ▶ ▶

See inside this helpcard for more information on how my illness can affect me and how you can help. ▶

Figure 1.6: Example of a help card

Most people prefer the support of family and friends rather than having to rely on professional carers. If family members and/or friends can work alongside the person with dementia to determine who can do what and when, it can make a huge difference to how supported the person with dementia feels.

Local community support

Local communities are about neighbours, and the wider community is about local organisations.

If people have supportive neighbours who are willing to keep a look out for them if they need help and to check on them regularly, that can provide a real sense of security.

Local community-based organisations may offer places to meet or to take part in activities. The list is endless but includes flower arranging, zumba, dancing, yoga, painting, gardening, etc. Many people will already have interests and local support can help to keep these going.

Professional support

A wide range of professionals can be involved in supporting people with dementia. Those who become involved will depend on the type of dementia and the level of support from family, friends and the community.

In all cases, the GP is likely to be a key person, along with a social worker who may have to agree a support plan. Specialist dementia advisors can also provide support, along with other professionals such as physiotherapists, speech and language therapists and professional carers, who provide additional support to that provided by family and friends.

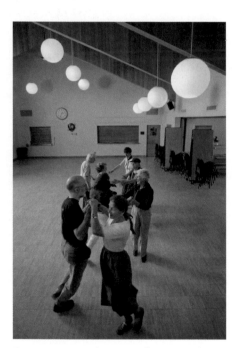

Dancing is one of a range of activities that may be supported through a community-based organisation.

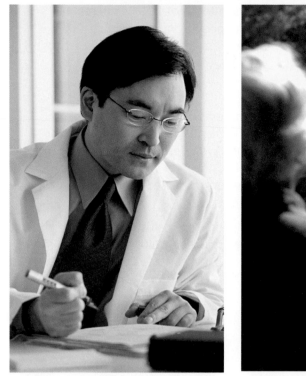

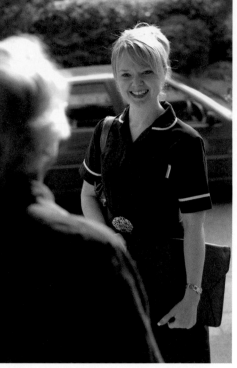

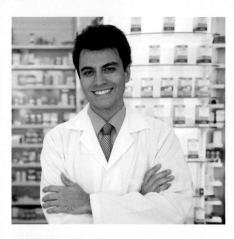

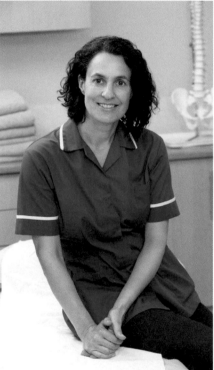

Have you had any dealings with pharmacists, GPs, occupational therapists or community nurses?

Assistive technology

There are continual advances in technology, and the way in which it is already being used to offer extra care and support is really helpful. For example, there are systems available that will monitor people's movements between rooms, so if they are wandering about at night, a carer can be alerted. There are systems that alert people if a door is left open, or if someone does not get out of bed, or if a person has a fall.

Health monitoring can also now be done using technology: this is called 'telehealth' as opposed to 'telecare'.

Age

The vast majority of people with dementia are over the age of 65.

The figures show that of the 750,000 people with dementia, over 16,000 are younger people. This means that they have 'early onset' dementia. The symptoms of dementia are similar, but the circumstances and the needs of younger people can be very different. For example, someone with early onset dementia may still be working, and wish to continue for as long as possible. They may still have dependent children and will be concerned about how to plan for their futures. They are likely to still be driving – this can continue for some time, but will need careful monitoring.

It is also often the case that younger people wait a long time for a diagnosis, as dementia is not an expected condition in younger people and can often be missed or misdiagnosed. Support from dementia services may not be as easy to access for younger people, as provision tends to be focused on older people. There may be age barriers, and there will often be barriers in terms of what is offered. For instance, activities may be arranged for older people and of no interest to someone younger. Younger people may have little in common with others using the services.

Type of dementia

Earlier in the chapter, we looked at the symptoms of the different types of dementia. The way that people experience dementia will be affected by their symptoms and the impact these have on their lives. Some people may find it hard to live with the frustration of struggling to find the right words for a conversation. Others may manage to live with that but be very distressed by the disorientation and fear of getting lost, and so stop going out.

The nature of the symptoms, coupled with people's circumstances and the amount of support they receive, means that everyone's experience of dementia is different and unique to them.

Case study

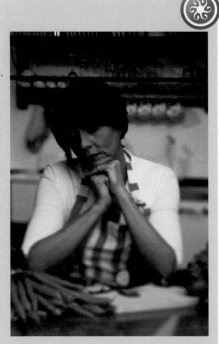

Sangeeta is 51. She works as a police officer. She is married with two children: one is at university and the other has just started A levels. Her husband works as an administrator for the local council. They have a mortgage which they increased recently in order to move to a bigger house and make some improvements.

Sangeeta has just been diagnosed with early onset Alzheimer's disease.

1   How do you think Sangeeta and her family will be feeling?
2   What issues will Sangeeta and her family have to think about?
3   What sort of support might they need?
4   Do you think there may be any problems with getting help?
5   If so, what would they be?

Activity

If Sangeeta lived in your area, what support would there be for her and her family?

Do some research and note down what is available in your area for someone like Sangeeta.

4.2 Attitudes and behaviours of others

There are many **stereotypes** about dementia. There is still a belief that it is a 'death sentence' and that people with dementia are not capable of living any sort of meaningful life. As one man with dementia put it, 'They seem to expect that we all sit around in chairs dribbling and are very surprised when we are not.'

An officer in charge at a day centre reported that a film crew had visited as part of a documentary, but had ended up not using the footage as it had not shown their expected view of people with dementia. They had simply filmed people having a good time, chatting to friends and being involved in activities.

There is an element of fear of dementia, partly as a result of the very term 'dementia' and its link to words like 'demented', but also because of lack of knowledge. The basis for all prejudice is fear and ignorance, both of which apply to dementia.

There is also a perception that people are no longer people when they have dementia. There are comments such as, 'She's no longer the person she was', or 'He's just a cabbage'. These types of comments show a huge lack of understanding of dementia and a failure to appreciate that *people are still people*. There may be some changes in how they relate to the rest of the world, but they are still the people they were before. It is our responsibility to work out how to relate to them.

Professional attitudes can be hugely varied. Some professionals view dementia as a medical condition that follows a pattern and has symptoms that need to be managed and reduced as far as possible. While treatment for the condition is important and correct diagnosis is vital, there is much more than this to supporting people with dementia. Professionals who stop short at medical interventions will help, but not as much as they could.

In later chapters we will look at how a person-centred approach to dementia can support people to live the best possible life while coping with their dementia. Professionals who are able to put *the person* at the centre of their work will offer the best possible experience for the person with dementia and their family.

> **Key term**
>
> **Stereotype** – a generalised, oversimplified view of a particular type of person or thing.

Getting ready for assessment

DEM 201 is a knowledge-based unit and each of the learning outcomes requires you to show your assessor that you have understood the learning. Your assessor may want you to do this through a written assignment or project, or you may be asked to prepare a presentation or undertake a computer-based task. Sometimes, assessors will check your understanding through a professional discussion where you will answer questions that demonstrate that you understand all the learning.

This unit is all about a broad introduction to dementia. It starts to cover several areas that are covered in more detail in other units. The first learning outcome is about the nature of dementia and what it is; you also need to understand the physical causes and effects of dementia. This unit requires you to show that you can

understand how dementia affects people and the impact it can have on their lives.

Your assessor will want to see that you have understood how a person's total environment affects their experience of dementia and that no two people's dementias are the same.

They will also want to see that you have understood how dementia is approached and the different models that are used to work with people with dementia.

When you are asked to 'explain' something, do not simply list or describe: use words and phrases such as 'because', 'as a result of', 'so that' and 'in order to'. If you are explaining something, you must show that you understand the reasons for it.

Further reading and research

- www.alzheimers.org.uk – Alzheimer's Society, the UK's leading care and research charity for individuals with dementia and those who care for them. The organisation provides information, support, guidance and referrals to other appropriate organisations.
- www.bild.org.uk – British Institute of Learning Disabilities, which works to improve the lives of individuals with disabilities. It provides a range of published and online information.
- www.cjdsupport.net – An organisation which supports individuals with prion diseases, including forms of Creutzfeldt-Jakob disease (CJD). They provide a range of information on the various forms of prion disease, and work with professionals to improve the level of care provided for individuals with these conditions.
- www.hda.org.uk – Huntington's Disease Association, an association that provides information, advice, support and useful publications for families affected by Huntington's disease in England and Wales. It can put you in touch with a regional advisor and your nearest branch or support group.

Chapter 2:
Person-centred approach to the care and support of people with dementia

This chapter covers the learning outcomes for units DEM 202 and DEM 204. DEM 202 is a knowledge unit, which underpins the competence that you will have to demonstrate in the workplace to achieve DEM 204.

Putting the person at the centre of your practice is an essential part of any work in social care, but when people have dementia it is even more important. It is easy to forget that *individuals with dementia are people*: professionals can sometimes respond only to the damaged brain and not to the personality and the human being that are still there.

Person-centred working is about looking at people's strengths – it involves working with what people can do rather than only looking at what they have lost. It is also about seeing the world from the perspective of the person with dementia. It is easy to forget that dementia makes the world seem a different place.

When you have achieved these units you will:

■ understand approaches that enable people with dementia to experience well-being
■ understand the role of carers in the care and support of people with dementia
■ understand the roles of others in the support of people with dementia
■ understand the importance of a person-centred approach to dementia care and support
■ be able to involve the person with dementia in planning and implementing their care and support using a person-centred approach
■ be able to involve carers and others in the care and support of people with dementia.

1: Understanding person-centred approaches

1.1 What is a person-centred approach?

Key values underpin work in this sector. These include:

- treating people as individuals
- supporting people to access their rights
- supporting people to exercise choice
- making sure that people have privacy if they want it
- supporting people to be as independent as possible
- treating people with dignity and respect
- recognising that working with people is a partnership, rather than a relationship controlled by professionals.

A person-centred approach is about recognising that everyone is different and has their own needs. Not everyone likes doing the same things, eating the same things, reading the same things or wearing the same things. Just because people have dementia and are making use of support and care services, it does not stop them from being a unique person with very particular needs.

Make sure that you do not make general assumptions about people. For example, not all older people like to play bingo or want to go out on coach trips. Some do and others do not. Not everyone wants to eat an evening meal at 5pm, or go to bed at 9pm, or get up at 7am. Some people do and others do not.

Ensuring that the key values listed above underpin the support for every individual is a vital part of a person-centred approach, but it is also about ensuring that support is centred on the whole person – not just the diseased brain. A person-centred approach focuses support on *abilities* rather than losses. It sees the person as a whole, taking into account important factors such as family, culture, ethnicity and gender.

Kitwood's model

Professor Tom Kitwood from the Bradford Dementia Group developed much of the thinking around person-centred approaches in dementia. He emphasised that it was important to maintain someone's 'personhood'. In other words, people should continue to be respected as individuals, with all the status that society recognised before they developed dementia.

Several studies have shown that if people continue to be treated with respect and valued for the abilities they still have, they benefit from increased self-esteem and well-being, and even show some improvement in dementia symptoms. This improvement is sometimes called **rementia**.

Kitwood showed dementia as an equation to support the view that it is not just about the disease and its effect on the brain. How each person experiences dementia is different depending on a range of factors in their lives.

Key term

Rementia – the improvement in dementia symptoms that can result from people being treated with respect and valued for the abilities they still have.

His view was that: **D = NI + PH + B + MSP**

D = dementia

NI = neurological impairment (the damage caused by dementia)

PH = physical health (the impact of illnesses, conditions or pain)

B = biography (a person's life history)

MSP = malignant social psychology (the negative ways that people with dementia are treated)

Kitwood's model is one way of trying to explain that how an individual's dementia develops, and the extent to which it affects them, is not just down to the development of the condition. It is also the result of their general health, their previous life experiences, and how they are treated by those around them.

Case studies

Susanna

Susanna has vascular dementia. She has lived alone in a high-rise flat for many years, but does not know any of the neighbours. Since she retired as a supervisor in a local factory, she has not been involved in many social activities. She used to go out with her sister, but since she died last year, Susanna has been very much alone. She was widowed 30 years ago and has no children. Her nieces and nephews hardly ever visit her. Susanna's health is poor, she has high blood pressure and her mobility is limited. Her dementia has progressed quite quickly and she is now unable to prepare meals or to work out how to get dressed. The last time she went to the shops, the police returned her home and referred her to Social Services. Susanna has now been assessed and will be going into residential care; she was judged not to have the capacity to make the decision about where she should live.

Saran

Saran has vascular dementia. He lives with his wife and his two sons and daughters-in-law along with four grandchildren. When Saran was diagnosed, his family researched vascular dementia and found out the best ways to support him. All the family, including the grandchildren, take turns to sit with him to talk or read to him and join in games and puzzles or to help him with painting, which he enjoys. His wife makes sure that he eats nutritious meals and he goes for a walk with a family member every day. His dementia is progressing quite slowly and he is still able to join in family discussions and to socialise with neighbours. Saran does not need any help with washing and dressing.

Sean

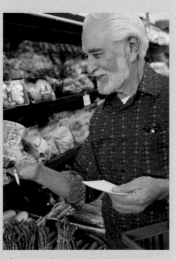

Sean lives alone in the same house where he was born. He has a mild learning disability and has lived alone for five years since his parents died. He knows most people in the local community and people always look out for him and make sure he is OK. The milkman always has a word and the local shopkeepers check that he hasn't forgotten any food items he needs. He goes to his next door neighbours every week for Sunday lunch. Sean has developed vascular dementia and has begun to be quite muddled about where he has left things and has forgotten to pay some bills and sometimes goes shopping twice. His neighbours and friends at the local pub have worked out a rota to check on Sean and remind him about things like paying bills and getting his shopping. They also have a rota to help him tidy up so it is easier to find things. Sean is coping well at the moment and does not have any help from Social Services.

Activity

Think about the differences in the three people in the case study. Make notes about how the different circumstances of each person makes their experience of dementia different. Now think about the people you support – what are the differences between them? How does this affect their dementia?

2: The importance of approaches to care and support that enable individuals with dementia to experience well-being

2.1 Benefits of person-centred working

Person-centred approaches do not just benefit the person with dementia. This way of working also provides significant benefits for the carers and/or family of the person with dementia, and for the professionals who are providing support.

Individuals being involved in their own care and support

The single most important benefit of a person-centred approach for the individual is that they are still treated as a person with wants and wishes and needs, not as a collection of symptoms to be managed.

The key value that underpins person-centred working is that *people with dementia are just people who sometimes get on with the world in a different way than they did before.*

A study by Tom Kitwood in 1995 and work by Elizabeth Barnett in 2000 showed that people who are given the right care and support can experience increased clarity of thinking (rementia). Their work shows the potential that people with dementia have to be able to function more fully if they are given the right kind of support.

There is also evidence from various research studies that the right care and support for people with dementia can:

• improve sleep patterns
• reduce agitation
• improve self-esteem
• improve quality of life.

In 1999, Burgener et al. worked with people in the early stages of dementia. They found that a person-centred approach involving the maintenance of activities that individuals had previously enjoyed resulted in positive quality of life outcomes.

Studies have shown that when people are given freedom of choice to manage their own lives and so have more say over things like mealtimes and activities, verbal agitation is reduced. This has also been found to have a positive effect on staff, who feel less rushed by not having to do everything for everyone at the same time.

Other work has demonstrated the positive effects of person-centred approaches on sleep patterns. Evidence has shown that when people are able to be involved in activities based on their previous interests and their current capability, daytime napping is reduced and night-time sleeping improves.

There are benefits to people's self-esteem when they are able to participate in planning their own support. This approach means that it is easier to focus on looking at what people *can* do, rather than on what they have lost.

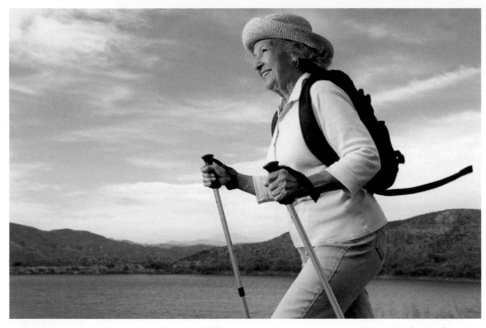

Why do you think a person-centred approach results in positive quality of life outcomes?

Making sure that the person with dementia is able to make it clear what support they want and how they want it to happen is often a challenge in terms of communication. In the next chapter, you will look at how to develop and use communication skills when working with people with dementia. There is no better place to use these skills than in supporting someone to plan their life and how they want to live.

There are also benefits to this approach for carers, whether family or professional. When people are respected and valued, they are likely to be more content and to feel that they have a better quality of life.

Reflect

Try to imagine how it feels to be unable to control your own life or to make your own choices. If you can, recall a time when that happened to you.

You may have been ill and felt that your treatment was being decided by others, or someone close to you may have been in that position.

It may have been a situation when you were much younger, at school or at home when you felt that you had no power to make any choices.

Try to remember how you felt in that situation. Were you angry or frustrated?

Think about how people with dementia must feel if they are not treated as a person worth listening to, or as someone who has a valid opinion.

How can you use this understanding to improve the way you work?

Involving people in planning and delivering their own support is one of the key ways of maintaining self-esteem. It shows them that they have an important contribution to make and have not been 'written off' because of a diagnosis of dementia. All of the research shows that people who are able to maintain self-esteem have better overall health and well-being, so the impact is very positive.

People planning their own lives and making choices can often mean that they will choose to take a far more risky path than social care professionals might have chosen. Everyone is entitled to take risks in order to be able to do the things that they want to do; professionals just need to have a positive approach to managing risks and to find ways to make it possible for people to exercise the choices they have made. There is more detail about managing risks in Chapter 5.

Using all you have learned about communicating with people who have dementia, you can support people to participate in planning their own support. There will be different levels of participation for people at different stages of the development of the dementia, but planning ahead and knowing what people want to happen in their lives is important, and helps them to feel more confident about the future.

Case study

Mary has Alzheimer's disease and is living in a residential unit.

She used to take a considerable amount of medication and spend much of the day sleeping in a chair in the lounge. In between sleeping, she would walk around shouting for 'George' and asking for someone to take her home. The pattern at night was similar, with episodes of wandering and shouting. Because of the disturbance caused to others, Mary was prescribed medication to improve her sleeping.

The whole approach of the residential unit changed following the appointment of a new officer in charge. Staff were trained in person-centred working and residents' medication was reviewed.

Staff spent time with Mary and her family to talk about her life. They discovered that she used to work in a multinational company as a personal secretary to a senior manager, and was a keen gardener in her spare time. Mary was able to contribute some of what she wanted: a plan was worked out where she would spend some time in the garden whenever she wanted, and would look after plants in her room. It was also agreed that one of the staff would keep an eye on the plants in case Mary forgot about them on some days. Mary's organising skills were also put to use: she offered as much help as she could to file the information that was being gathered for a project about the history of the local community. This was being planned with pupils from a local school.

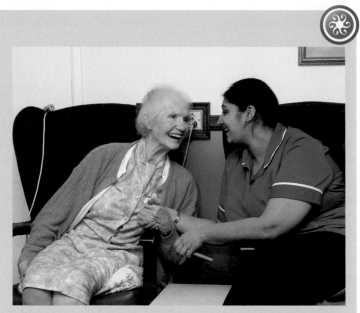

When Mary stopped taking so much medication, she was much more alert in the daytime. Her activity in the garden and working on the local community project made her quite tired, so she began to sleep better. She was far less agitated because someone would always respond to her as soon as she began to worry about wanting to go home.

1   What difference did a person-centred approach make to Mary?
2   What do you think may have been the future for Mary without the change in approach?

3: Working with carers in the care and support of individuals with dementia

3.1 The role of carers

The 2001 census identified that there were six million carers in the UK: 12 per cent of the adult population. The increasing number of older people, along with the policy of empowering people to remain active in the community for longer, means that the number of carers is forecast to rise by over 50 per cent to almost nine and a half million by 2037, less than 30 years away. Not all these carers are supporting someone with dementia, but very large numbers are.

Carers are a vitally important part of a support plan for a person with dementia. Most people who care do so willingly and lovingly, but this does not mean that the role is easy or without serious demands and a great deal of stress.

Carers have a vital role in working in partnership with professional staff. The balance of the care delivered will vary, and may change over time. Initially, family carers may be providing most of the support, perhaps with some extra professional support. As dementia progresses, it may be that the person is cared for, in the main, by professional staff, with family or friends offering additional care support when needed. A key element of the person-centred plan is the role played by family or friend carers.

Family and friend carers are often the best people to support communication with the person with dementia, as they are likely to know them best and to understand their needs. They will also know the person's history and be able to help professional staff to research a full individual history. A family carer can sometimes be the best person to calm and reassure someone if they are agitated and distressed, and they can often be very helpful in working out the causes of distress or anxiety.

There are two very different scenarios for carers:

1. When a person with dementia remains in their own home, or the home of the carer, and they are supported by professional staff. This situation still leaves the carer feeling in control and able to continue caring for their loved one in their own way. This means that their role is clear and well understood – they are in charge of providing the necessary support for the person with dementia and the professional care staff are supporting them in their caring role. In this situation, a person-centred plan should be able to identify the specific areas in which the person with dementia or their carer needs support. All other aspects of the person's life are for them to decide on, with the support of their carer(s).

In these circumstances a carer's role can range from popping in occasionally to ensure that the person has managed to undertake all their daily tasks, to carrying out a full-time supporting role. If a carer is a partner, their role is likely to develop gradually as the dementia progresses. It may start as just reminding or checking, and then grow to the point where they are providing 24-hour care.

2. When a person with dementia is in residential care, and it is difficult for carers to find the right balance between working with professional staff and seeing that they still have a role. When someone goes into residential care, a carer's emotions can be very mixed. Some people may feel very guilty that they have been unable to continue to care for their relative at home, but this may

Why is Scenario 1 so positive for carers?

also be coupled with relief at no longer having the responsibility. This confusion of emotions can sometimes make it difficult for carers to work with professional staff initially. It can give rise to situations where former carers can criticise and complain about the work and standards of professional staff. Alternatively, carers can sometimes disappear and believe that they have no useful role to play.

Above all, it is important to recognise that former carers are still the people with the best knowledge and understanding of the person with dementia.

Activity

Think about a person you support who has a family or friend carer. Make some notes about how they are involved in the support and planning for their loved one.

Think of at least three further ways in which they could be involved and work in partnership with you.

If you do not support anyone who has, or had, a family or friend carer, ask a colleague about someone they have worked with.

AC 204:3.2

3.2 Involving carers

Tell me and I'll forget, show me and I may remember, involve me and I'll understand.

Chinese proverb

Case study

Yolanda has dementia. She is 75 years old and was cared for by her daughter, Sherece, until her memory lapses meant that she was placing herself and her daughter's children at risk: by leaving heaters and cookers on, and by leaving the door wide open at night.

Following Yolanda's admission to residential care, her daughter is keen to be as involved as possible in her mother's support package. In the planning meeting it is agreed with Yolanda that her daughter will come and share lunch with her most days and will then stay for a couple of hours each afternoon.

Yolanda is interested in music: she used to sing in the local choir and played the piano. One afternoon each week, Sherece takes her to a local music group for people with dementia and other memory issues, where people can play instruments, listen to music and reminisce. Another afternoon, Yolanda likes to bake. Sherece helps her to remember the recipes and to bake in the residents' kitchen.

Sherece agrees to maintain responsibility for checking that Yolanda's medication is in the locked cupboard in her room.

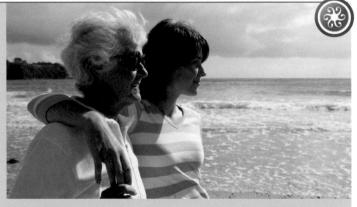

The staff have trained her in how to administer medication and Sherece understands the responsibilities of the Registered Manager. She continues to collect Yolanda's repeat prescriptions and to check that her mother has taken her tablets each day when she arrives.

What are the benefits of Sherece being actively involved in her mother's support plan:

1 for Yolanda?
2 for Sherece?
3 for the professional staff?

Involving carers as partners in the support of a person with dementia is the best way for them to understand person-centred working. This means them doing as much as they want to in relation to caring for their friend or relative: just because someone is now in residential care does not mean that friends and family carers are no longer needed or important. It just means that they no longer have to do all of the caring alone.

There are various ways of involving carers. Much will depend on the wishes of the person with dementia and the extent to which a carer is prepared to work in partnership with professional staff. There is no reason why a family or friend carer cannot continue to be involved with many aspects of an individual's personal care if they both wish it. Or it may be preferable that they are involved in social activities or in creative tasks.

Not all carers may want to be as actively involved as Sherece in the case study, and some may want more. For many people, being fully involved in planning and decision making is the most important aspect of care. In a person-centred approach, this goes beyond consultation: it means real involvement and a voice in all decisions. It also means that carers must be prepared to work in a person-centred way and to support the person with dementia to make as many of their own choices as possible.

3.3 Increasing carers' understanding of dementia and a person-centred approach

AC 204:3.1

You may find that carers understand dementia better than you do! Many carers will take a great deal of time and effort to understand the condition that has affected their loved one. Of course, not all will do so, and not all will think about it with a person-centred approach.

Carers do not always find it easy to let go of choices and control of a person's life. Families may want to protect people who they see as vulnerable and in need of care. They may have many concerns about increasing the independence of loved ones who have dementia, who may be taking risks in order to do the things they want. Do not jump to the conclusion that families are being difficult or obstructive. Usually, people believe that they are doing their best for their relatives by protecting them and by reducing risk.

Working in partnership with people and their families to help them get used to new approaches, and to see the benefits of person-centred approaches, may be a slow process that needs to be taken gently. The long-term benefits of people being able to maintain as much control as possible over their lives is worth the effort.

Ways of sharing information with carers

Many carers find it helpful to understand the processes of dementia and exactly what happens as the condition progresses. This may have been explained by doctors and dementia nurses, but it is always worth checking that people have understood the explanations.

Useful information is available through various organisations (see *Further reading and research* in Chapter 3). If carers have access to the Internet, they can take part in forums involving other carers and relatives.

Supporting carers to understand the type of dementia that their loved one has, and the likely progression path, will help them to recognise the different stages of the condition and to be ready for changes as they happen. It will also help them to prepare for changes and to be ready to adapt to meet different needs.

People take in information in different ways, so make sure you find out individuals' preferences. Some people like you to sit and talk to them. Others prefer written information that they can take away, look at in their own time and then come back with questions. Some people may want you to recommend websites where they can research for themselves. Others may want to be put in touch with other carers who are in a similar position.

Communicating with carers

The rules about effective communication are just as important for carers as for the person with dementia. Remember the basics, such as finding out about:

- preferred methods of communication
- preferred language
- preferred format
- specific communication needs.

Explaining about person-centred approaches and making sure that carers are supportive of this way of working can be something of a challenge. For many carers, though, the concept is something that they have already been doing. They may well have been ensuring that their loved one is able to make choices and to participate as an equal partner. If this is the case, they will welcome any residential facility or domiciliary support service that works in this way.

A straightforward way to explain the concept of person-centred working is to say that it is *the difference between people having to fit into the services that are available and the services having to fit the people who want to use them.*

It is also important to explain the idea of the *whole person* rather than just thinking about the dementia. It is valuable for carers to understand that everything about a person's history and life, along with the attitudes of others, has an impact on how they will cope with their dementia. It can also be helpful for carers to understand that person-centred work focuses on what people *can* do rather than the things that they can no longer do.

3.4 Developing a professional working relationship with carers

The first national strategy for carers, Caring for carers, was introduced in 1999. Since April 2001, carers have had further rights under a new law: the Carers and Disabled Children Act 2000. This entitles carers to an assessment of their needs if they wish. This can be done when the person they care for is being assessed, or separately. The carer can, with guidance from a social worker or care manager, assess themselves.

The Carers (Equal Opportunities) Act 2004 came into force in England on 1 April, 2005. The Act gives carers new rights to information and ensures that work, lifelong learning and leisure are considered when a carer is assessed. The Work and Families Act 2006 extends the right of carers to request flexible working.

Some situations require much more than words of support. Giving practical, physical support to a carer or family may help to make it easier for them to manage their caring responsibilities.

The extra support provided by a professional carer can do this in two ways:

1 It can provide the additional help which allows the carer to feel that they are not in a hopeless, never-ending situation.

2 It can provide an opportunity to encourage carers to think about themselves and their needs.

Carers' rights and benefits

Carers' assessments

Carers have the right to have their needs assessed by Social Services regardless of whether the person with dementia has also had an assessment.

These assessments are an important way of finding out what support carers may need. They should cover:

- how people feel about their caring role, e.g. do they love to do it, find it a burden, find it frustrating?
- whether the carer is coping with the level of care they are currently providing, and how this may change in the future
- what help a carer may need to be able to carry on providing care
- whether caring is affecting the carer's health
- whether the carer is able to enjoy any leisure interests
- whether the carer wants to work, or to access training
- the contingency plans that need to be put in place for an emergency if the carer is suddenly unable to continue to provide care.

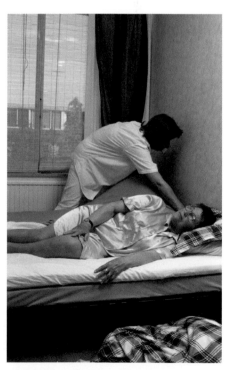

What do you think are the advantages and disadvantages of having a professional carer or a family/friend carer?

Activity

Think about any people you support who have family or friend carers. Ask if they are willing to tell you if they have had a carer's assessment. If they have, find out what services they were offered as a result.

As in the earlier activity on page 34, if you do not support anyone who has, or had, a family or friend carer, ask a colleague about someone they have worked with.

Your local Social Services department should have information in its performance review about how many carers' assessments have been carried out in your area.

1 Find out from your local carers' support organisation how many carers are in your area.

2 How do the numbers of assessments carried out match up to the numbers of carers?

Benefits and support available to carers

Carers are entitled to various financial benefits. One of your roles in supporting carers is to check that they are aware of the benefits available to them and that they are claiming everything they should.

You are not expected to be a welfare rights expert. However, being able to give carers information about where to get advice is useful, as is having a broad knowledge of benefits for carers.

Benefits that may be available are:

- Carer's Allowance (certain conditions apply)
- Income Support (for carers under pension age)
- Pension Credit (for carers who are pensioners)
- Carer Premium (paid on top of other benefits)
- National Insurance contributions (paid for every week someone is providing care: this protects the carer's pension).

There are detailed conditions for all of these benefits: it is important to advise carers to seek expert advice if they think they are not getting all the benefits they should be.

Table 2.1 shows examples of the types of support that can be made available to carers.

Table 2.1: Examples of support that can be provided for carers

Situation	Solution
Carer needs to be able to take breaks when necessary.	Either regular or flexible breaks can be arranged. Some areas operate voucher schemes so that carers can organise breaks when it suits them. Others have regular planned breaks.
Carer needs aids, equipment and adaptations.	The physical environment can be adapted to make caring easier, e.g. hoists, ramps, accessible bathrooms and electronic aids can all make the caring task easier.
Carer needs support to work or undertake training.	Carers can be provided with support for the cared-for person while they are at work, and they can be helped to undertake training courses in order to return to work.
Carer needs some time and interests for themselves.	Carers can be provided with support while they are involved in a leisure activity. Advice and information about opportunities, as well as practical support, is available from a range of sources, e.g. the Internet, local library.

Activity

Research the main benefits and support available for carers, based on the information in this section. You can find information online or by visiting your local library or Citizens Advice Bureau.

When you have collected all the relevant information, write it up into a table so that you can refer to it easily.

Vulnerable carers

Never forget that sometimes the carer can be just as vulnerable as the person with dementia, particularly if the person's behaviour is challenging.

For example, if a partner is caring for someone with dementia who exhibits challenging behaviour, the partner may be very much at risk. It is important to look at the *whole* picture when looking at a risk assessment, and to offer support and protection to any vulnerable adult who is at risk.

Case study

Maggie is 75 years old. She is quite fit, although increasingly her arthritis is slowing her down and making her less steady on her feet.

She is looking after Guy, her husband, who has dementia. He has communication difficulties: he struggles to recall the words he wants to say. His ability to complete daily tasks such as getting dressed is limited, e.g. he has problems with buttons, shoelaces and what garments to wear. Guy also suffers from major mood swings and can be aggressive.

Maggie is his only carer. She does visit the GP regularly, but does not have any other help – her husband's mood swings make it difficult and sometimes he refuses to have people in the house.

Recently, Maggie has had an increasing number of injuries. In the past two months she has had a grazed forehead, a black eye and a split lip. Last week, she arrived at the GP surgery with a bruised and sprained wrist. She finally admitted to the GP that Guy had inflicted the injuries during his periods of bad temper. She said that these were becoming more frequent as he became more frustrated with her slowness.

Despite being very distressed, Maggie will not agree to being separated from Guy. She is adamant that he does not mean to hurt her. She will not consider residential care.

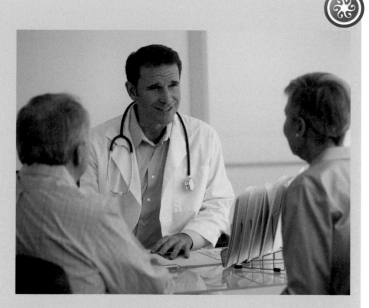

Finally, Maggie agrees to have some assistance with daily living, provided that her husband does not get too angry.

1 What action can be taken?

2 What action *should* be taken?

3 Who has responsibility for this situation?

This kind of situation may cause a great deal of concern and anxiety for families and professionals. However, there are limits on the legal powers to intervene, and there is no justification for removing Maggie's right to make her own decisions.

Activity

Imagine that you are the support worker for Guy and Maggie. Your work involves regular visits to their house to monitor the effectiveness of the care package and to provide support. One day you arrive to find Guy screaming at his wife and hitting her.

1 What would your immediate actions be?

2 Write a report covering the incident, including your actions.

3 To whom would you give the report?

4 Who else would need to be informed of this incident?

Professional working relationships with carers are important for:

- the person with dementia
- the carer
- the professionals.

The person with dementia benefits because they are able to maintain a relationship with someone who is dear to them and an important part of their life. Even if they do not appear to be aware of the person any more or to recognise them, they will benefit and take comfort from having a family or friend carer involved in their life.

Professional working relationships with carers are important for the carers because they are able to be involved and supportive to the person they care about. They are also able to have their support valued and recognised. This is vital – whether they are caring for someone in the community, or working in partnership with professional staff in residential care.

The professionals also benefit from professional working relationships with carers, because carers know the individual best and can give valuable information about someone's history and background. They are also likely to understand reasons for some behaviour, or be able to suggest reasons for particular anxieties or worries.

If the person you are supporting is able to maintain close contact with a family or friend carer, the person will be happier and their overall well-being is likely to improve.

■ **Learning outcome**
204:2

AC 204:2.1

4: Involving the person with dementia in their care and support using a person-centred approach

4.1 Personality and life history

The key thing that life histories do is to change the views of people around the person with dementia. Family or friend carers are likely to know the person well and still be able to see them as they were. The difficulty for professional care and support staff is that it is easy to only see the person who is in front of them now. It may be hard, without finding out about a person's history, to be able to see beyond that.

If someone has quite advanced dementia, it can be difficult to see their personality. There may be occasional moments where you see a sense of humour, or a real skill, but generally it is not always obvious beneath the symptoms of the dementia. Finding out about a life history can almost 'bring someone back' and help to understand the person who is still there.

If you know about the events in a person's life, it makes reminiscence work much easier: you can be sure that you are touching on areas of real interest that are likely to spark recollections and conversation. Knowing about the work that a person did, or the interests and hobbies that they had, can help when you are working with them to plan activities.

It is important that once a life history is complete, it is used to improve a person's well-being and to help them live with dementia. As discussed earlier, being involved in activities that are of interest to a person with dementia has been shown to improve their well-being: through better sleep patterns, less daytime napping and a reduction in agitation and anxiety. All of these outcomes help to improve a person's quality of life.

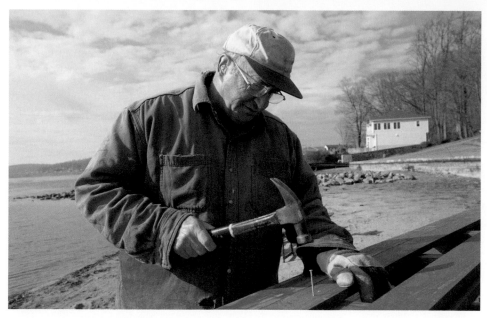

Finding out about someone's past hobbies and interests can give you a better idea of their personality.

You will learn more details about the importance of life history, and about how to find out and record the details of a person's life, in Chapter 3.

Reflect

The list of interesting aspects of any person's life is very long.

Think of one person that you support.

Make notes about what you really know about them and how much you understand about their life:

- What sort of person were they: the life and soul of the party, or quiet and shy?
- What was their job? Were they thought to be very good at it? What were their achievements?
- What about interests and hobbies, and family and friends?

Now think of one person you know well – perhaps a parent, sibling or other relative, or maybe a lifelong friend.

Make notes under the same headings about how much you know about them. You will probably be surprised at how much you know.

Imagine that you were the carer for your relative or friend. Consider how much information you could share with professional carers, how much it would help them to know and understand the real person who is hidden behind the dementia.

The information that you obtain in order to compile a life history can be invaluable in many aspects of work with someone with dementia. With the person's (or their advocate's) agreement, relevant parts of the information can be shared with others who are working with them. For example, GPs, physiotherapists, community nurses or occupational therapists may all be able to develop more effective approaches if they have an understanding of the person's life history.

4.2 Communication

You must feel confident that you are able to use a range of methods and means of communication, depending on the needs of the person you are supporting.

Alzheimer Europe suggests one framework for approaching and communicating with someone with dementia: the 'Ten Commandments'. These are split into two categories, as follows.

Doing it well

Approaching the person with dementia

1 Stand close to the person.
2 Use the person's name regularly.
3 Touch the person's body.
4 Stand at the person's height and face to face.
5 Establish eye-to-eye contact.

Communicating with the person with dementia

1 Speak slowly and clearly.
2 Use short, simple, clear and concrete words and sentences.
3 Complete your words with gestures and touch.
4 Give one message at a time.
5 Use affirmative sentences.

Source: adapted from Alzheimer Belgium (www.alzheimer.be)

The 'Commandments' are a useful set of guidelines to follow in all communication with people with dementia. They are particularly relevant to verbal communication. It is important not to argue with someone who has dementia. It is better to respond in a non-committal but positive – affirmative – way.

For example, if someone says that she needs to get home for tea or her mother will worry, try to look beyond the *words* that the person is using. Perhaps she may mean that she is feeling insecure, lonely, scared or vulnerable.

Communication can be in many different forms, depending on the person's needs and preferences. For someone with advanced dementia who may no longer use verbal communication, you may need to use non-verbal gestures, facial expressions and touch.

Just because people no longer talk does not mean that they have no wish or need to communicate. Picture cards can be useful, or sometimes people will draw, or model, or build messages out of objects around them. Someone who constantly collects objects may be expressing anxiety, or may just be reverting to behaviour from many years ago when they were, for example, tidying up after their children.

Doing it well

When you are working with people with dementia, these are important points to remember about communication:

- Find out how people prefer to communicate.
- Be prepared to use all forms of communication.
- See the whole person, not just the dementia.
- Never take behaviour at face value.

You will learn more about the importance of communication with people with dementia, and how the ability to communicate is affected by dementia, in Chapter 3.

Do not forget that **behaviour is a means of communication**. Think carefully about what someone is communicating through the way they are behaving.

4.3 Identifying and managing risks

Everyone is entitled to take risks.

We all take risks in our daily lives: every time we get on an aeroplane, cross the road, put money in a bank, take part in a sporting activity, plug in a toaster, etc. We assess these kinds of risk and make sure that they are managed. For example, we know that there are stringent safety procedures in place for aircraft, we look left and right before we cross the road, we know that there are regulations in place for banks, we take steps to maintain electrical safety in our houses, etc.

So, taking risks is part of being able to choose and be in control of your life. With this in mind, it is important to make sure that concern about risks is not getting in the way of people with dementia living their lives in the way they want to. Often, a **risk assessment** can make it possible for someone to do something that may seem unlikely in the first instance, as the case study below illustrates.

Person-centred approaches put people with dementia at the centre of everything. They look at what people *can* do and identify what they want to achieve.

Sometimes the things that people may want to achieve will involve risks. This is not a problem as long as they are not actually putting themselves in danger, or there are ways of reducing the risks in potentially 'dangerous' activities.

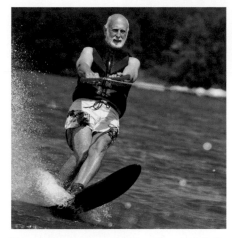

Would you regard this as too risky?

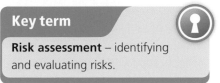

Key term

Risk assessment – identifying and evaluating risks.

Case study

Sam has been diagnosed with dementia. He wants to stay living in his own home where he has been for the past 50 years.

His son and daughter are very concerned: they both live some distance away and are convinced that their father should go into residential care, as they believe he will be at risk if he remains living on his own.

A risk assessment looks at ways of reducing the risks to Sam of staying at home. The assessment may look at the steps that can be taken for Sam to maintain his independence in the way he wants to. There could be regular drop-ins from a support worker, and a link set up with a local supported living unit where Sam could go if he feels he needs support. It may also be possible to install telecare equipment that will monitor Sam and contact a call centre if there are concerns such as appliances left on, or the door left open.

With Sam's agreement, neighbours and friends in the local community can help with watching out for him and checking that he is all right, or offer assistance if he gets lost or confused.

With all the steps in place to reduce the risks, it makes it possible for the son and daughter, who are concerned for Sam's safety

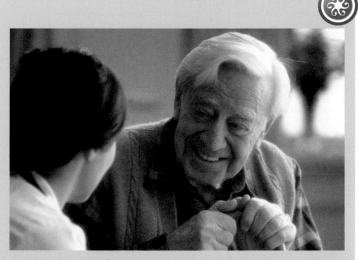

and well-being, to feel more confident. It also means that Sam can continue to have the benefits of living somewhere he is comfortable and familiar, in a neighbourhood he knows and is known.

1   What are the risks to Sam?
2   What else could be done to reduce these risks?
3   Who has the final say in this situation?
4   What are the benefits to Sam of staying in his own home?

Some people may need to be encouraged to take some risks. This is shown in Henry's case study.

Henry is 75. He used to be very active and a keen runner, despite having a visual impairment caused by macular degeneration, and having been diagnosed with Alzheimer's disease.

As he got older, Henry always walked for at least a mile each day, regardless of the weather.

One day he got lost on his way home from the library. He was very distressed and was brought home by a neighbour. After this, he was very reluctant to continue walking each day: he and his wife both felt it was too risky and so stayed indoors. This made him very depressed and put a strain on his relationship with his wife.

Their support worker spoke to both of them about being prepared to take some risks in order to support Henry to get back to his daily exercise. Initially, the support worker went with Henry each day and they made a note of the

key landmarks on the routes he usually walked: Henry kept the notes in his pocket. As Henry felt more confident, the support worker gradually reduced her support, although Henry's wife would often go with him and found that she enjoyed the exercise too.

After a couple of months, Henry was back to his usual daily walks. He carried a note in his pocket with his address and contact numbers, along with the landmarks he knew he needed to look out for. Henry was able to continue his walks for many months before his condition deteriorated.

1   Why was it important for Henry to continue walking?
2   Do you think it was right to encourage Henry to continue walking? Why?

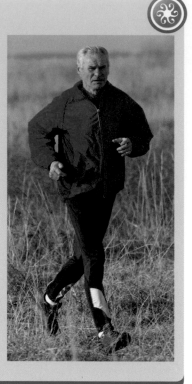

AC 204:2.3

4.4 Taking opportunities that meet agreed abilities, needs and preferences

Life does not have to be over because of a diagnosis of dementia: there are still so many things that people can do.

Person-centred approaches mean always looking for what people *can* do rather than what they can no longer do. Taking time to communicate with a person with dementia about opportunities, and finding out about things they really want to do, is a constructive use of time, and is likely to result in improved well-being for the person.

There are many different opportunities that people may want to follow up, depending on their own interests and the current stage of their dementia. It is vital that, wherever possible, they should be opportunities that *the person* has identified as being something they are interested in and want to do. If this is not possible, perhaps because someone is in the later stages of dementia, it should be opportunities that are known to be areas of interest, and that are making best use of the person's abilities.

What people can do depends largely on the stage of their dementia and the impact it has had. Dementia is different for everyone and people will retain different abilities for differing lengths of time.

Table 2.2 shows the kinds of opportunities that people with dementia may want to experience, and the effects of dementia and support required when considering each type of opportunity.

Table 2.2: The possible effects of dementia and support required for a range of opportunities

Opportunity	Effects of dementia	Ideas for support
Physical exercise, e.g. walking, swimming, dancing	*Early stages*: possibly loss of confidence, so may need encouragement — to continue alone if at all possible *Later stages*: possibly disorientation, memory loss and increasing frailty	*Early stages*: maps, address and key landmarks *Later stages*: exercise/activity may be shorter and accompanied, but change of scene and/or fresh air are important
Team games and activities; board games/any activity with rules	*Early stages*: difficulty remembering rules, shorter concentration span, language/communication difficulties, issues with making choices	*Early stages*: may need reminders of rules, longer time to participate
Art/craft activities	Lack of memory and concentration will indicate the need for simpler activities without complex patterns to follow	May need encouragement and reminders
Puzzles, crosswords	Language and memory loss Reduced concentration/focus	May need some assistance and reminders Offer short puzzles, or undertake activity in short sessions
Reminiscence, memory boxes, photos: one-to-one or in a group	Language and communication, reduced concentration	May need time to communicate (simple yes/no questions are better); encourage family or friend carers to participate
Day-to-day activities: dusting, food preparation, sweeping, gardening, etc.	Understanding and processing information	Instructions need to be simple and short
Sensory activities: music, reading aloud, views, fish tank, massage, scented oils	*Later stages*: helpful to offer sensory stimulation; senses are not usually directly affected by dementia	

The important thing is that opportunities should be something that the person with dementia enjoys and wants to participate in.

Depression and lack of motivation can often be part of dementia, and so people may need encouragement to take up opportunities. Once motivated, their well-being should improve as they are involved in something stimulating and enjoyable.

5: The roles of others in the support of people with dementia

5.1 The roles of other professionals involved in care and support

There are many different people whose professional roles can involve support for people with dementia.

Not all of them will be involved with every person with dementia, but everyone with dementia is likely to have a team of professionals offering support. Table 2.3 shows the main types of professional involved with people with dementia, and their roles.

Table 2.3: The role of professionals who support people with dementia

Professional	Role
Care and support worker	Personal care, assistance with daily living, physical and emotional support (at home or in a residential setting)
Social worker	Assessment, review, safeguarding, risk management, support package, therapeutic support, group work, re-ablement
Physiotherapist	Exercise and mobility: preventive or following injury/illness
Consultant specialist	Expert medical support specialising in dementia: diagnosis, prescription of any medication and treatment plan
Psychologist	Dealing with emotional issues: interpreting behaviour
Manager	Overall responsibility for residential/nursing home or domiciliary care: ensures quality and reliability of service delivery
Occupational therapist (OT)	Development activities to maintain health and well-being
GP	Medical support for health and well-being: e.g. repeat prescriptions, arranging community health support
Speech and language therapist (SLT)	Support for communication and language
Pharmacist	Dispenses medication, provides advice on minor illnesses
Nurse	Provides health support in the community
Independent mental capacity advocate (IMCA)	Represents the best interests of the person with dementia
Community psychiatric nurse (CPN)	Monitors and treats mental health issues in the community
Dementia care advisor	Expertise in all aspects of dementia and care: supports the person with dementia and their carers
Advocate	Represents the views of the person with dementia
Support group	Can provide the chance to meet with others who have dementia and share experiences and concerns; there are also groups for carers

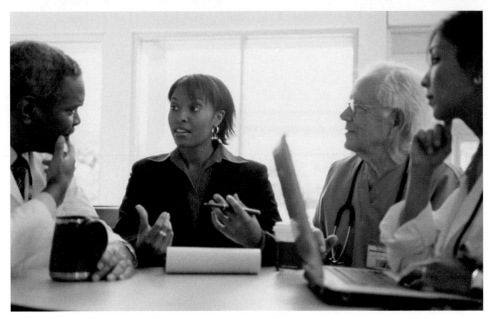

How many different professionals work with the people you support?

It is important that you understand what other professionals do so that you are able to refer to them for support if necessary, and to explain to people with dementia and their families how they can gain access to support if they wish to.

5.2 Making referrals

AC 202:3.2

Your role in supporting someone with dementia is vital and it covers many of their needs. However, you cannot do everything, and some areas of work require a very high level of skill and training.

For example, if someone is having mobility problems as a result of their dementia, or due to arthritis, or perhaps a fall or an injury, then a physiotherapist will be able to help by prescribing appropriate exercises. You will be able to help by assisting the person with dementia to do the exercises given by the physiotherapist.

During the diagnosis of dementia, a consultant who specialises in dementia is likely to be involved. They will make the diagnosis and will prescribe necessary medication. They will also monitor the progress of an individual's dementia and will amend treatments as necessary.

A diagnosis of dementia can be very traumatic for a person and their family. A dementia care advisor supports people through this stage. They provide all the necessary advice and guidance to help people and their families come to terms with how their lives will change, and how they can make changes and adaptations in order to live positively with dementia.

If someone has reached the later stages of dementia and no longer has the capacity to make their own decisions, an independent mental capacity advocate can be appointed to ensure that the person's interests are represented.

5.3 How to access the support of others

AC 202:3.3

Making a referral to gain the right support for someone is part of your duty of care as a professional. It is important that you are able to recognise when and how to do this. Most referrals are made either through the social worker or through the GP. They will then contact the relevant professional and arrange for an assessment.

Activity

Look again at the list of professionals in Table 2.3.

1 For each one, note down the circumstances where you might make a referral.
2 Then research how you would contact each of them. Would you contact them:
   - directly?
   - through the GP?
   - through the social worker?
   - through another route?

Getting ready for assessment

DEM 202 is a knowledge-based unit and each of the learning outcomes requires you to show your assessor that you have understood the learning. Your assessor may want you to do this through a written assignment or project, or you may be asked to prepare a presentation or undertake a computer-based task. Sometimes, assessors will check your understanding through a professional discussion where you will answer questions that demonstrate that you understand all the learning.

This unit is all about person-centred approaches, so you will have to show that you understand why person-centred approaches are important, and how they put people in control of their lives.

Your assessor will want to see that you have understood how person-centred approaches look positively at dementia and ocus on what people are able to do, rather than what they cannot achieve.

They will also want to see that you have understood how risks can be used positively in order to support people to be in control and make choices about their lives.

DEM 204 is a competence-based unit that focuses on knowledge and demonstration of skills. You will need to demonstrate in a workplace setting that you are able to involve people with dementia and their carers and families in their own support.

This means that you must show that people have chosen their own support package as far as possible, and that families and friends have also been involved.

You need to have found out as much as possible about the person you are supporting and know how their history influences their present. Your assessor will want to see that you have used life history to help you to understand a person's behaviour.

As with DEM 202, you must show through your work that you are focusing on the positive aspects of people's abilities, and offering opportunities that make the most of what people are able to do.

When you are asked to 'explain' something, do not simply list or describe: use words and phrases such as 'because', 'as a result of', 'so that' and 'in order to'. If you are explaining something, you must show that you understand the reasons for it.

Further reading and research

Skills for Care: Common Core Principles for Working With Carers (www.skillsforcare.org.uk).

Chapter 3: Communication and interaction with individuals who have dementia

This chapter covers the learning outcomes for units DEM 205 and DEM 210. DEM 205 is a knowledge unit, which underpins the competence that you will have to demonstrate in the workplace to achieve DEM 210.

One of the hardest consequences of having dementia is that people can become very isolated. They may find it difficult to communicate and so stop trying. Just at the time when someone's life is becoming confusing and quite frightening, more and more people seem to stop making contact with them. Take a moment to imagine how that must feel.

There are many ways to communicate with people, regardless of the challenges they may be facing. It is a question of thinking in a different way and working out how the world looks from the point of view of the person with dementia. Once you can do that, their behaviour can make much more sense.

These units are vital: they underpin everything you do to support people with dementia. If you are not communicating well, you are not doing your job.

When you have achieved these units you will:

- understand the factors that can influence communication and interaction with individuals who have dementia
- understand how a person-centred approach may be used to encourage positive communication with individuals with dementia
- understand the factors which can affect interactions with individuals with dementia
- be able to communicate with individuals with dementia
- be able to apply interaction and communication approaches with individuals with dementia.

1: Factors that can influence communication and interaction

> It is important not to assume that people with Alzheimer's disease have lost understanding or knowledge. It is too easy to think that they do not know simply because they do not communicate. We need to take on the challenge of finding ways to communicate successfully, to try different routes to find common ground.
>
> *Professor Trevor Harley, University of Dundee*

AC 205:1.1

1.1 Effects of dementia on communication and interaction

Everyone has their own experience of dementia. It is not the same for everyone and so much depends on the progress of the condition, the living environment and the physical condition of each individual. You can learn about the possible effects of dementia on communication and interaction with others, but not everyone will have the same experience. The progress of dementia will have an impact on each individual that will be unique to them.

Remember also that dementia is not a single condition, it is a term used to describe the symptoms of a range of conditions. If you think back to Chapter 1, you will recall that different conditions cause people to develop different symptoms, but most people with dementia will experience the isolation of increasing difficulties with communication.

Symptoms can cause various difficulties for people with dementia. Some people 'write off' someone with dementia and assume that it is not possible to communicate with them, or give up at the first hurdle and do not bother to try other options if they get no response the first time they try.

Dementia frightens many people. They do not understand it, and some have preconceptions that it makes people 'mad' or dangerous. Understanding dementia is the first step towards removing fear and to making it more likely that people

Reflect

The main difficulty relating to communication and interaction with people who have dementia is the negative attitude of people who do not understand dementia.

The world of someone with dementia is a different place than it used to be. It is confusing, sometimes frightening. It is certainly frustrating and can be very sad. To work well with people with dementia, it is important to think about how their world looks, and to respond to communication from their point of view. Do you always do this? Or do you try to make a person with dementia adapt to the ways you want to communicate with them?

To help you reflect on the way you interact with people with dementia, think about this quotation from Professor Tom Kitwood, who has been one of the pioneers of person-centred work in this field:

'As we discover the person who has dementia we also discover something of ourselves. For what we have ultimately to offer is not technical expertise but ordinary faculties raised to a higher level: our power to feel, to give, to stand in the shoes (or sit in the chair) of another.'

Kitwood, T. (1993) 'Discover the person, not the disease', *Journal of Dementia Care* 1(6) 16–17

with dementia are accepted and recognised as being part of communities, neighbourhoods, families and friendship groups.

The symptoms of dementia *do* have an impact on how people communicate:

- It can be difficult to find the right word for something they want to say.
- They may repeat something they have already said several times.
- They may be confused about where they are or what time period they are in.

All of these effects can make communication difficult, but it is certainly not impossible.

Verbal communication

For many people with dementia, finding the right words can be a struggle. Words can be lost completely, or just take time to remember. People can also use the wrong word so that a sentence does not make sense.

It is easy to feel that there is no point in trying to continue a conversation, but it is important to carry on: to make every effort to understand and to make yourself understood. Difficulties with finding words, or using the wrong words, can cause great frustration, especially when the person may not realise that they have the wrong word. They may repeat it, often getting increasingly irate because the listener is not understanding. Sometimes people with dementia will speak quite fluently, but the content does not make sense to those listening.

When people become disorientated about where they are in place and/or in time, it can have a significant impact on language and spoken communication.

Think about how many words you use in ordinary speech that are related to time and place. Table 3.1 provides some examples.

Table 3.1: Words commonly used in conversations relating to time and place

Place	Time
Here	When
There	Now
Where	Then
Over there	Before
Over here	After
Going	Later
Coming	Soon
Been	This year/week/month
	Next year/week/month
	Today/tomorrow/yesterday

Activity

Try to add to Table 3.1 with other examples of everyday words that you use which are related to time and place.

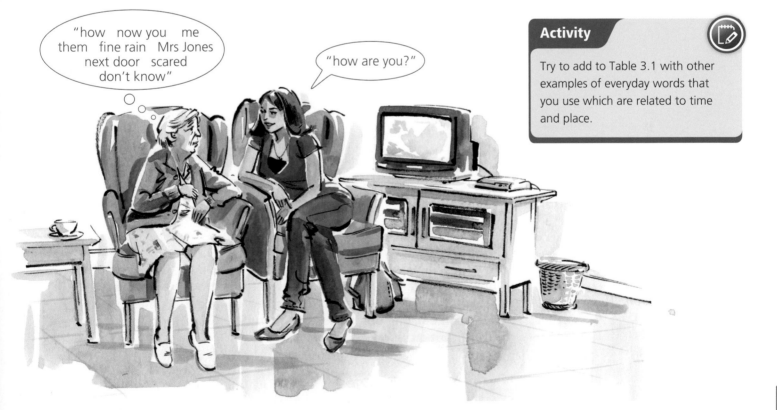

Figure 3.1: Verbal communication can be a big challenge for a person with dementia.

As you think of words you use all the time, consider how hard it would be to communicate and interact with others if none of the words meant the same thing to you as it did to them.

When someone is unsure about where they are or what year it is, some – or all – of the time, you can see how hard it must be for them to communicate and interact with others. If people are unsure of where they are, then much of what they say may be inappropriate. If they are confused about what stage of their life they are in, they may make comments that make no sense to someone who is clear about the here and now.

Written communication

Writing is a skill that can often be lost by people with dementia.

To be able to write requires a complex range of skills, such as:

- recognising the symbols and letters that make words
- having the motor coordination to transfer the words to paper or screen
- an ongoing review of what you are writing to ensure that it is communicating what you want.

In the same way, reading is a complex mix of skills, which requires:

- sufficient eyesight to see what you are reading
- the ability to recognise the symbols and letters in front of you
- brain processes to translate what you can see into a communication that can be understood.

The reduction in the ability of the brain to process information can often result in people with dementia struggling to make sense of the written word.

However, this is not true of everyone. For some people with dementia, writing becomes a useful way of expressing themselves. Powerful books and poems have been written by people with dementia: some of these are included in Further reading at the end of the chapter.

Non-verbal communication

Non-verbal communication is probably the most important way of communicating and interacting with people with dementia.

You may remember from your previous learning about communication that only 7 per cent of our communication is through words: the remaining 93 per cent is through non-verbal communication.

> **Dementia sufferers seem sometimes to have a heightened awareness of body language, and often their main meanings may be conveyed nonverbally. In the case of those who are very severely impaired it seems probable that the words and sentences are at times more of an accompaniment or adornment than the vehicle for carrying the significant message.**
>
> **(Tom Kitwood, 1993)**

One of the effects of dementia for some people is that the world feels like a confusing and frightening place. A touch or a kind smile can make a big difference: it can help to reassure someone who is uncertain. As dementia symptoms progress and people are increasingly affected in different areas of their lives, their ability to communicate reduces – or changes – significantly. Being able to recognise and respond to these changes is the sign of a good professional care worker who makes a real, positive difference to the lives of people with dementia.

As people lose the ability to use language, or to process the words they hear from others, they communicate more through non-verbal means. Close observation of facial expressions, movements and gestures is vital to support communication and reduce the sense of isolation experienced by people as their dementia progresses.

Non-verbal communication covers many ways of communicating, for example:

- facial expressions
- eye contact
- tone of voice and the loudness or softness of speech
- how fast or slowly people speak
- touch and physical contact
- body posture and movement
- gestures
- body distance and closeness
- dress, appearance and smell
- use of the environment and objects to get a message across
- creative activity, including sculpture, music, painting, dance and movement.

Creative activity can be a useful means of expression for many people. It can provide them with a means to communicate using a range of art forms, including those listed above.

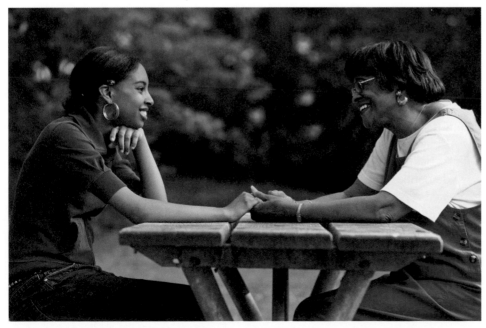

Non-verbal communication is vital to support verbal communication.

The impact of dementia can close down many aspects of people's lives. However, professional social care staff can support people to develop new ways of communicating and maintaining a connection with those around them.

1.2 Other factors that influence communication and interaction

History

People who develop dementia do not suddenly become different people. They still have the same background, upbringing and history that they have always had, and they still have many of the same personality traits that they have always had. Sometimes people with frontal or temporal lobe dementia may undergo a personality change, but for many people their familiar characteristics will still be there. So someone who has always struggled to communicate, who has been very shy and lacked confidence, is likely to still be reluctant to take the lead in conversations. Someone who has always been chatty may still try to reach out and communicate with others, even though the ability to use language in the same way may be less evident.

The work people have done may also be a clue to communication. For example, someone who has had a senior job and may be used to giving orders and telling people what to do may still try to do that. One man with dementia would constantly repeat numbers: it was discovered that he had worked in an abattoir and used to count the animals in. Someone who has been a teacher may repeat, 'Be quiet!' or 'Sit down!', as if they are talking to a class of children.

Physical conditions and pain

Conditions such as a hearing or visual impairment can affect how people with dementia communicate. When people have dementia it is easy to assume that all communication issues are due to the dementia, and to forget that other factors may play a part. Hearing or vision problems can be overlooked: hearing or eye tests may not happen, and hearing aid batteries and glasses may not be checked.

A stroke can result in communication issues similar to those experienced by people with dementia. Following a stroke, people can find it difficult to use language and may take time to process communication from others.

Pain is a major issue for people who have dementia. A study carried out for the Alzheimer's Society found that, following hip replacement surgery, patients with Alzheimer's were given 53 per cent less pain relief than people who did not have dementia. There appears to be a view among medical staff that pain not expressed is pain not felt. Pain can be difficult for a person with dementia to express or explain. They may not be able to process pain messages to understand the cause of their discomfort, and so may find it hard to communicate that they are in pain.

Pain can be the result of a range of conditions, including:

- arthritis
- constipation
- dental problems – badly fitting dentures

- urinary tract infections
- pressure ulcers
- tight or uncomfortable clothing
- headaches – wrong prescription glasses
- undiagnosed fractures.

Pain can cause reduced concentration, increased memory loss, increased confusion, aggressive behaviour, sleep disturbance or depression. All of these factors have an effect on a person's ability to communicate and to interact with people around them.

Case study

Kassim has Alzheimer's disease and is in a nursing home. His dementia is quite advanced and he has almost completely stopped using language to communicate. Over the past few weeks he has become increasingly agitated and keeps repeating, 'Help me – help me!' and moving his head from side to side. He seems to be getting more confused and is becoming very unsettled at night. There have been discussions about using anti-psychotic medication or stronger sedation.

A new care assistant noticed that Kassim was eating very little. She was concerned and checked on him over a couple of days. She noticed that he seemed to be fine with soup and he would eat fish, but always left meat and vegetables. The only desserts he ate were jelly and ice cream. She also noticed that his teeth seemed to be slipping as he was eating his meals.

When Kassim's mouth was checked it was discovered that he had several large mouth ulcers where his dentures had been rubbing. As the dementia progressed and he had lost weight, his dentures had become too large for him and the damage had gone unnoticed.

A visit to the dentist and treatment for the mouth ulcers cleared up the problem. As a result, Kassim was much less agitated. He

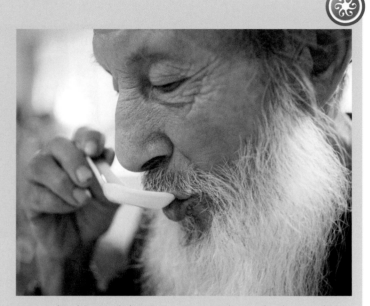

returned to his usual sleeping pattern and went back to smiling at everyone – and enjoying his meals.

1 What could have prevented this situation?
2 Why do you think Kassim's condition was not noticed?
3 What could have happened if no one had discovered the issue with Kassim's dentures and the mouth ulcers?

Mental health

Depression and anxiety can be symptoms of dementia. Both of these conditions will have an effect on how people are able to respond to others.

Depression makes it very hard for people to have an interest in making conversation or to respond to others. Concentration is reduced and poor sleeping patterns can make memory loss and confusion worse.

Anxiety can also affect concentration. People can become very distressed as they constantly seek reassurance, making any other communication or interaction very difficult.

Key term

Anxiety – feelings of nervousness, worry or unease.

Environmental factors

Do not forget what you have learned about how environmental factors can affect communication.

Environmental factors apply as much to people with dementia as anyone else:

- Noisy rooms can make it hard for people to concentrate.
- Being too hot or too cold can also affect concentration.
- Rooms where others are talking, where the television is on or music playing can make it hard to hear.
- If someone has the sun in their eyes, it can make concentration and communication difficult.

Doing it well

When looking at communication in people with dementia, it is important to think past the dementia.

Look at all possible factors that affect people's communication, regardless of whether or not they have dementia. As we have discussed in this section, these factors include:

- their history
- physical conditions and pain
- mental health
- environmental factors.

AC 205:1.3 and 210:1.1

1.3 Memory impairment and the use of verbal language

Memory

Our memories are quite amazing and perform the most complex and challenging processes.

Despite plenty of research, there is still no certainty about how or why memory works as it does. The most widely held view is that there are three important functions of memory:

1 **Encoding** – this means receiving and processing information.
2 **Storage** – this is about keeping the information somewhere it can be found if needed.
3 **Retrieval** – this is the process of recalling information as and when it is needed.

In order to carry out these complex tasks, we all have different sorts of memory:

- **Sensory memory** is a very short memory, literally milliseconds. We use it when we first see or hear something. It is this memory that means we can look at something and remember how it looks or what it sounds like.
- **Short-term memory** contains information that we can remember and recall for short periods of time, usually up to half a minute.

- **Long-term memory** is infinite in size and can store and recall information over very long periods of time, sometimes over a whole lifetime. All memories stored for longer than 30 seconds are in the long-term memory.

The long- and short-term memory process and store information in different ways, using different parts of the brain:

- The frontal lobe is involved in short-term memory.
- The temporal lobe and cerebellum are important for long-term memory.
- The hippocampus moves information from the short-term to the long-term memory.

Long-term memory

The key parts to the long-term memory are the **episodic** and **semantic** memory.

Episodic memory

The episodic memory holds information about events or 'episodes' in a person's life. The episodic memory holds them in three main ways:

- **Explicit memory** is used when we consciously recall events and previous experiences. This means you can remember your holiday or where you were yesterday, or an event when you were at school.
- **Implicit memory** is when you are not aware of using this part of your memory. It is used to recall information that you use in day-to-day activities without being aware of recalling it. You use implicit memory to do things like brush your teeth, tie a shoelace or drive a car.
- **Procedural memory** is used to store information about skills like making a cake, painting a wall, repairing a car or making a meal.

Semantic memory

This part of your memory holds information, facts and figures, and part of it stores words. We use semantic memory to recall factual information. When you respond to quiz questions, you raid your semantic memory for the answers.

The part of the semantic memory that stores words is affected in dementia, which is why people with dementia sometimes struggle to recall the right word to use.

Effects of memory loss

As the different parts of the brain are affected during the progress of dementia, memory function is lost or reduced. Usually, short-term memory is affected most significantly, whereas people are able to recall many areas of long-term memory.

Unfortunately, it is the short-term memory that is used to deal with experiences in the present. In order to hold a conversation, you have to be able to remember what has just been said so that you can reply. In order to read a sentence in a book or newspaper, you need to be able to remember the first part of the sentence to make sense of the ending.

Language is something we all acquire in childhood. There are many different theories about how humans develop language, but broadly it begins at around six months with 'babbling'. It continues over the next few years as a learning process until we are fully able to communicate with others. The reason that we are able to use written or verbal language to communicate is because the information about

> **Key terms**
>
> **Episodic memory** – this holds information about events or 'episodes' in a person's life.
> **Semantic memory** – this holds information, facts and figures, and part of it stores words.

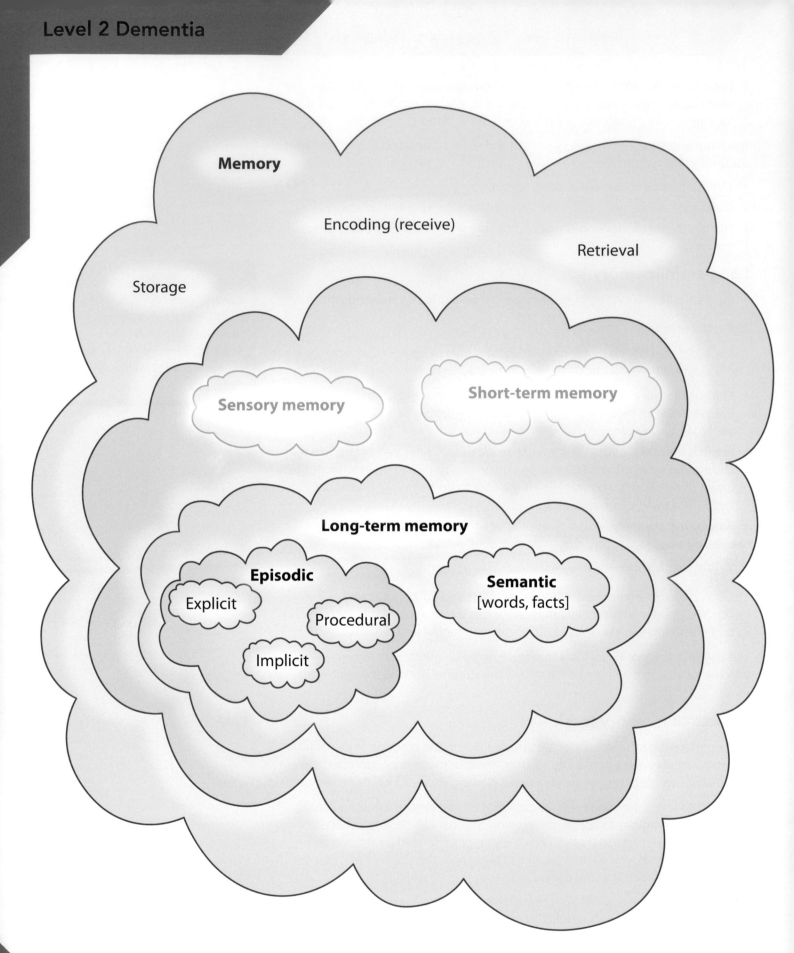

Figure 3.2: Functions and types of memory

how to use language is stored in our memories and we are able to recall it in order to use it.

The development of dementia can damage the parts of the brain that remember the language we need to use and the right way to use it. It is important to recognise that not all parts of memory will be lost as dementia progresses, and memory will be lost at different rates. This means that people can be supported to adapt and use the memory functions that they have in order to help communication.

Activity

- Look at ten objects on a tray for ten seconds. Then try to recall as many of them as you can.
- Try again five minutes later.
- Next, look at an old school photograph. Try to remember the names of as many people as possible.

When you initially look at the ten objects on a tray, you are likely to be able to recall between four and seven items. This is your short-term memory. When you try again five minutes later, you will probably recall fewer items than you could originally.

You will probably recall far more names from the photograph than you could of the objects you looked at. This is because it is your long-term memory that is being used to recall the information. As touched on above, it has an infinite storage capacity and can recall over a much longer period of time.

You will probably recall more names the longer you keep looking at the photograph and try to remember, whereas your short-term recall is likely to decrease after a short period.

2: How a person-centred approach can encourage positive interaction and communication

■ **Learning outcomes**
205:2, 210:1 and 210:2

2.1 Identifying communication strengths and abilities

AC 205:2.1, 210:1.3 and 210:1.4

Person-centred approach

As discussed in previous chapters, a person-centred approach is all about putting the individual at the centre of everything you do. Instead of making them fit into the system, you adapt and change the system to meet their needs.

This applies as much to communication as to every other aspect of the support you provide. One of the consequences of developing dementia is that people stop being treated as a *person*: they can lose their **personhood**. The concept of personhood is about all the essential things that make someone who they are. Professor Tom Kitwood described it as 'a standing or status that is bestowed upon one human being by others in the context of relationship and social being, implying recognition, respect and trust'.

Key term

Personhood – all the essential things that make someone who they are – a status that recognises individuals in society.

If the focus is on the diseased brain and the losses of memory and function, rather than on the positive aspects of the whole person, then that person is devalued and loses their status as a person.

Recognising strengths and abilities

Recognising the abilities and strengths that people have, rather than what they have lost, is the key to supporting them to communicate well and make good relationships with those around them.

We are all different in terms of how we communicate and which methods suit us best. Everyone has their own way of communicating that is unique to them: you will communicate differently from your colleagues, friends and members of your family. Some people are very good at meeting people and talking. Others find meeting strangers a nightmare. Some people write letters, articles or reports extremely well, and others struggle to put a few sentences together. There are people who are more comfortable giving someone a hug or holding their hand than trying to find the right words.

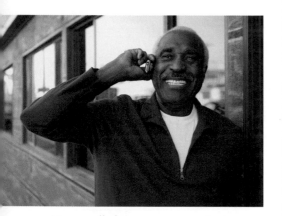

How well do you communicate on the telephone?

> ### Activity
>
> Rearrange the following activities in your order of preference, Number 1 being something that you enjoy and are very comfortable doing, Number 10 being something that you would dread, or feel unable to do.
>
> 1 Give a presentation to a group of about 30 people.
> 2 Have a chat with a friend over coffee.
> 3 Go to a party where you only know the host.
> 4 Ask a question in a staff meeting in front of six colleagues.
> 5 Write an article about your job for a staff magazine.
> 6 Telephone someone you have never met to make a complaint.
> 7 Paint a recognisable picture of someone you know.
> 8 Talk to someone who has just been bereaved.
> 9 Put your arm around someone who is upset.
> 10 Go with a partner to a dinner party with three other couples you have never met before.
>
> What does this activity tell you about your strengths and abilities when it comes to communication?

Understanding unique needs and preferences

Everyone has things they are good at and things they are not so good at: developing dementia does not always change all of that.

As dementia develops and different functions are affected, the skills that people retain will vary, but they are the key to successful communication. For example, some people may communicate better through touch and facial expressions if they struggle to find the right words. Others may still be able to find words, but may lose track of a conversation, so are good with very short interactions. Some people may have great ability in written communication, or even drawing, and this can be very useful as a means of communication.

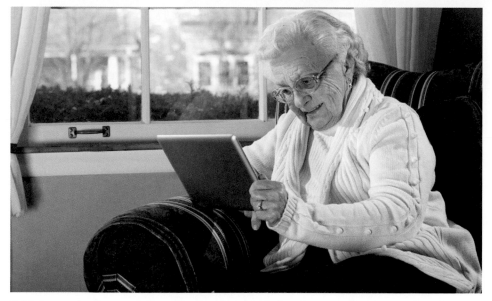

Which are the best communication methods for the people you support?

Getting information

AC 210:1.2

The best ways to find out about the strengths that people have are by asking and observing. Take notice of what people respond to and work out how they like to communicate and what they are good at.

Gathering information from other people who are involved is also an essential part of ensuring that you have it right. There are many people you can ask for information, with the permission of the individual of course. They could include:

- family
- friends
- professional colleagues
- GP
- district nurse
- day centre
- pharmacist
- advocate
- speech and language therapist.

Doing it well

Other people will have different experiences of interacting with the person, so they should be able to give you valuable information.

When asking for information, remember the following:

- Gain the agreement of the person, wherever possible.
- Explain to the person you are asking why you want the information.
- Only ask for the information you need.
- Record any information you are given so that it does not have to be found a second time.

2.2 Adapting communication styles to meet needs, strengths and abilities

We all have a style of communicating that is our usual way of interacting with the world around us.

Some people are noisy and chatty, others are quiet and calm. Some people are very tactile and make a lot of physical contact with others, some are more reserved and use touch very rarely. There are very mobile and active people who use many different facial and body movements, such as waving their hands around, while others are very still and hardly move, and have very little facial expression.

We are all different.

Reflect

Either watch a recording of yourself interacting with others, or ask a friend or colleague to observe you and note down your style of communication.

In the light of what you have seen or read, think about your style of communication and how you present yourself to others.

- Do you respond to the needs of others and change your style in order to meet their needs?
- Or do you always come across in the same way?

Consider what you could do to make sure that you are sensitive to the needs of the people you support.

Assuming that you have already found out about people's communication abilities, you need to consider how you can best use a person's strengths to make it easier for them to enjoy interacting with you.

Verbal communication

For many people with dementia, a spoken conversation is still how they like to communicate. As people progress into the later stages of dementia, they may be less likely to take the initiative and start a conversation, so you may need to be the one who gets the ball rolling.

If you are using verbal communication, you may need to make some changes to your preferred style.

Here are some examples:

- If you are usually a person who speaks quickly, you will need to slow down, but not so much that it becomes difficult to follow – just slower than you usually speak.
- If you are inclined to ask lots of questions, you need to make sure that you ask one at a time, and leave plenty of time for the person to process what you are saying.
- Use very simple, closed questions that only need a 'yes' or 'no' answer.
- Avoid long, complicated sentences with interrelated ideas. For instance, do not say, 'It's getting near tea time now, isn't it? How about some tea? Have you

thought about what you would like?' Instead say, 'Are you hungry? Would you like fish? Would you like chicken?', and so on, until you have established what sort of meal the person wants.

- If you have a loud voice, or tend to shout, think about speaking in a calm way with an even tone. Loud voices or an aggressive sounding tone can cause people to become agitated and distressed.

In summary, use very simple, short sentences, speak slowly and be prepared to wait while the person processes what you have said and composes a reply.

Non-verbal communication

Touch

Using touch can be helpful, so if you are someone who does not tend to make physical contact, you may need to adapt your preferred style. Touch can be reassuring and helps people with dementia to get the sense of your meaning, even if they cannot follow every word.

Body language

In the same way, body language can convey much of the meaning of what you want to communicate, and people can usually read body language very well. If you do not usually think about your body language, try to become more aware of it. Use gestures: they make it easier for people to understand the idea that you are trying to get across.

Words and pictures

Many people with dementia have good skills in recognising written words and in using pictures. This can be a valuable way of adapting communication so that people can get the most benefit from using their abilities to interact through visual, rather than spoken, means. Drawing, writing or using flash cards can be a very helpful means of communication for a person with dementia.

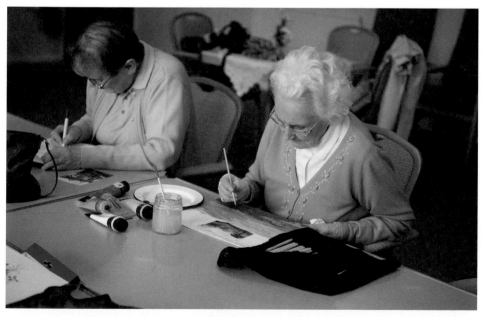

Painting and drawing can be valuable forms of interaction and communication.

Listening

Regardless of the means or method of communication, listening is one of the most important communication skills. You should listen well whether you are 'listening' to spoken words, body language, written words or pictures.

Specific adaptations

Some people have communication issues in addition to dementia. These issues may include:

* hearing loss
* visual impairment
* learning disabilities: these are quite common as there is a high incidence of young onset dementia among people with Down's syndrome
* physical disabilities that may require a different style of communication, for example, for someone who has had a stroke or who has a condition such as Parkinson's disease.

Hearing loss

When you are working with someone who has a hearing loss, ensure that any means of improving hearing which the person uses, such as a hearing aid, is:

* working properly
* fitted correctly
* installed with fresh, working batteries
* clean
* doing its job properly in terms of improving the person's hearing.

Make sure that you are sitting in a good light, not too far away from the person. Speak clearly, but do not shout. Shouting simply distorts your face and makes it more difficult for a person with hearing loss to be able to read what you are saying. Some people lip read, while others will use a form of sign language for understanding. This may be BSL (British Sign Language) or Makaton (which uses signs and symbols). The individual may rely on a combination of lip reading and gestures.

Remember that, as dementia progresses, people may struggle to communicate using signing or gestures, as recalling the signs and gestures becomes more difficult.

Visual impairment

One of the most common ways of assisting people who have visual impairment is to provide them with glasses or contact lenses. Make sure that they are clean and that they are the correct prescription.

Let people know that they should have their eyes tested every two years and regularly update their glasses or lenses. A person whose eyesight and requirements for glasses have changed will have difficulty in picking up many of the non-verbal signals that are part of communication. Someone with dementia may well forget about updating their glasses, or may even forget to put them on.

Dementia can cause problems with depth perception or recognising objects. Use of contrasting colours can help with this, as can having similar colours in flooring so that people do not 'see' a step where none exists. This is covered in more depth when we look at a person's environment in Chapter 5.

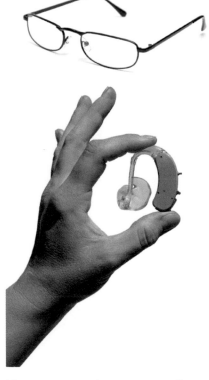

How can you adapt your care for a person with dementia who has hearing loss and/or visual impairment?

Let someone with a significant visual impairment know that you are there by touching and saying hello, rather than suddenly beginning to speak and 'arriving' unexpectedly. When you do start talking, make sure that you introduce yourself, for instance, by saying, 'Hello John, it's Sue.'

You may need to use touch more than you would in speaking to a sighted person, because the concerns that you will be expressing through your face and your general body movements will not be seen. For example, if you are expressing concern or sympathy, it may be appropriate to touch someone's hand or arm at the same time as saying you are concerned and sympathetic.

Having a visual impairment can make the progression of dementia even more frightening and confusing. Being able to maintain communication and interaction is of vital importance.

Physical disabilities

Physical disabilities or illnesses have to be dealt with according to the nature of the disability.

Conditions such as cerebral palsy can lead to difficulties in speech, although not in comprehension. Depending on the stage of the dementia, the person will understand perfectly what you are saying but they may have difficulty in communicating with you. You will have to be prepared to allow additional time for a response, due to the difficulties that the person may have in producing words, as well as the processing difficulties as a result of the dementia.

You may also have to become familiar with the sound of a person's voice and the way in which they communicate. It can be hard to understand people who have illnesses that affect their facial, throat or larynx muscles. The person may have been provided with assistive technology that enables them to communicate by producing an electronic 'voice'. However, technology can become difficult to operate as dementia progresses.

Learning disabilities

You need to adjust your methods of communicating to take account of the level of learning disability that a person has. You should have gathered sufficient information about the individual to know the level of understanding that they

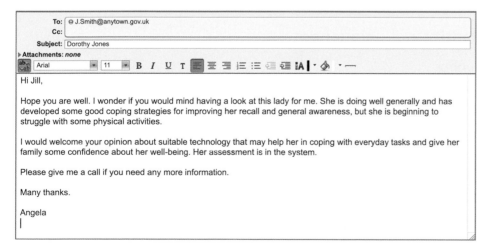

Figure 3.3: Technology may be able to help those with physical disabilities as well as those caring for them.

have: how simply and how often you need to explain things, and the sorts of communication that are likely to be the most effective.

Some people with a learning disability respond well to physical contact. They are able to relate and communicate on a physical level more easily than on a verbal level. This will vary between individuals and you must find out the preferred means of communication for the person you are supporting.

> **Doing it well**
>
> Here are some ways that you can adapt your communication styles:
>
> - *Loud, quick speech* → speech that is slower, calmer, with an even tone.
> - *Complex questions (several questions together)* → ask one question at a time; ask closed questions that require simple 'yes' or 'no' answers; leave plenty of time for answers.
> - *Reserved, very little touching* → use touch to reassure.
> - *Not much expression or body movement* → use facial expressions, gestures and body movement to help get the message across.
> - *Written communication only* → write single words, upper case first and then lower case, e.g. 'Tea', 'Biscuit', 'Medicine'; draw a simple, single item on each piece of paper or card.

AC 205:2.3 and 210:2.3

2.3 The importance of the identity and uniqueness of an individual

We are all individuals. Working in a person-centred way recognises and values each person for what and who they are. One of the problems with traditional approaches to dementia is that the individual gets lost and that they are only seen in terms of the damage that is being done by the dementia. All of the aspects of their lives disappear as they become a set of symptoms: their personality, sense of humour, achievements, kindnesses and family life can all be lost.

Person-centred approaches mean that people are valued for who they are and that all the important things about them are still there.

Identity and uniqueness

Identity

Identity or **self-image** is about how people see themselves.

How would you describe yourself?

- Is it in terms of what you do – for example, a support worker?
- Is it in terms of your relationships with others – for example, as a wife, a parent or a child?
- Is it as someone's mum or daughter?
- Is it in terms of your hopes, dreams or ambitions?

Or perhaps it is more likely that all of these ways of thinking about you play some part.

> **Key term**
>
> **Self-image** (or self-concept) – how people see themselves.

Think about the number of different ways you could describe yourself. List them all.

Check how many relate to:

- other people, for example, as someone's mum, sister, friend
- what you do, for example, care worker, volunteer at the youth club, gardener
- your beliefs, for example, honesty, loyalty, Christianity, the Muslim faith
- what you look like, for example, short brown hair, blue eyes.

You may be surprised when you see the greatest influences on how you view yourself.

Identity is what makes people who they are. Everyone has an image of themselves: it can be a positive image overall or a negative one, but a great many factors contribute to a person's sense of identity.

These factors include:

- gender
- race
- language
- religion
- environment
- family
- friends
- culture
- values and beliefs
- sexuality.

Uniqueness

All of these factors are aspects of our lives that contribute towards our idea of who we are. As a support worker, it is essential that you take time to consider how each of the people you work with have developed their own self-image and identity, and it is important that you recognise and promote this. Just because someone has dementia does not mean that all of this has disappeared and been lost. It is just as important as it was before the dementia developed.

Make sure that you recognise that the values, beliefs, tastes and preferences that people have are what define them. They must be supported, nurtured and encouraged, not ignored and disregarded because they are inconvenient, or do not fit in with the care system, or do not seem to matter because someone has dementia.

Reflect

Focus on one person with dementia with whom you have worked.

Note down all the influences on their sense of identity. Have you really thought about them before?

Think about the difference it may make to your practice now that you have spent some time reflecting on the influences that have made the person who they are.

Recognising everyone as unique is reinforced by knowing about how they prefer to communicate, and what their strengths and skills are. The fact that you have asked others for information and taken time to find out about an individual shows that you are putting them at the centre of your practice.

The information you have gathered will help you to plan the best means of using someone's strengths to support their communication. This means that they are not being required to fit into your approach, but that you are going to adapt your practice to accommodate their needs.

■ **Learning outcomes**
205:3 and 210:2

AC 205:3.1 and 210:2.2

3: Understanding and applying approaches to interaction and communication

3.1 How to use biography and history to facilitate positive interactions

The importance of life history

If you are going to work with someone, it is important that you know as much about them as possible.

You have looked at ways of finding out information about people. There are various ways of doing this, but the most effective is always to ask the person concerned whatever you want to know. Try to find time to sit down with the person and ask them about their life. Someone with dementia will usually be able to recall much of their earlier life. If they are able to tell you about their own history you will learn a great deal, and it will help you to offer support in the most appropriate ways.

It is often easy to think about people, especially older people, as you see them now, and to forget that their lives may have been very different in the past. The following poem is said to have been found in the early 1970s in the locker of a geriatric patient, Kate, after her death.

> *What do you see, nurses, what do you see?*
> *What are you thinking when you look at me?*
> *A crabbit old woman, not very wise,*
> *Uncertain of habit with far-away eyes*
> *Who dribbles her food and makes no reply*
> *When you say in a loud voice, 'I do wish you'd try'*
> *Who seems not to notice the things that you do*
> *And forever is losing a stick or a shoe*
> *Who, unresisting or not, lets you do as you will,*
> *With bathing and feeding – the long day to fill.*
> *Is that what you're thinking? Is that what you see?*
> *Then open your eyes nurse – you're looking at me.*
> *I'll tell you who I am as I sit here so still*
> *As I rise at your bidding, as I eat at your will.*
> *I'm a small child of ten with a father and mother*
> *Brothers and sisters who love one another,*
> *A young girl of sixteen with wings on her feet*

Dreaming that soon a lover she'll meet
A bride soon, at twenty my heart gives a leap
Remembering the vows that I promised to keep.
At twenty-five now I have young of my own
Who need me to build a secure happy home
A young woman of thirty, my young now grow fast
Bound to each other with ties that should last.
At forty my young ones have grown and are gone
But my man stays beside me to see I don't mourn
At fifty, once more babies play round my knee
Again, we know children, my loved one and me.
Dark days are upon me as my husband is dead
I look at the future, I shudder with dread
For my young are all busy rearing young of their own
And I think of the years and the love I have known.
I'm an old woman now and nature is cruel
'Tis her jest to make old age look like a fool.
The body it crumbles, grace and vigour depart
There is now a stone where I once had a heart.
But inside this old carcass a young girl still dwells
And now and again my battered heart swells.
I remember the joys, I remember the pain
And I'm loving and living life over again
I think of the years – all too few – gone too fast
And accept the stark fact that nothing can last
So open your eyes, nurses, open and see
Not a crabbit old woman… look closer, see ME.

Reflect

This poem demonstrates clearly how easy it is to forget that everyone has a history: that people's lives will have been very different from their present circumstances.

Can you think of a time when you may have forgotten this? Think about the people you support and be honest about how much you know about them. Do you really know about their history, such as what sort of lives they had, when they fell in love, got married, had children, what times were like then?

If you realise that you do not know enough about the history of the people you support, now is the time to change and start to ask questions. You may be surprised at the interesting lives people have had, and about how much they have done.

Depending on the stage of dementia, you may not be able to get all the background history you are looking for from the person concerned. If the person gives their consent (if they are able to), family and friends will be the best source of information, if they are willing to share it.

Putting together a life history

Putting together a history of someone's life is a fascinating activity. It will really help you to see them as a whole person, not just the person with dementia whom you know now. There are many different ways to put together a life history. If you can do it alongside the person, it can be valuable in terms of providing a base for reminiscence work and for improving concentration and memory.

Life story book

You may want to create a life story book, containing photographs and information. This is particularly good if there are family members who can participate and provide photographs and memories to complete the book: it is a good activity for families to do together.

Chart with a timeline

A life history can also be done as a chart, with a timeline showing the key dates of major life events, such as when someone:

- was born
- went to school
- left school
- started work
- fought in the war
- got married
- had children.

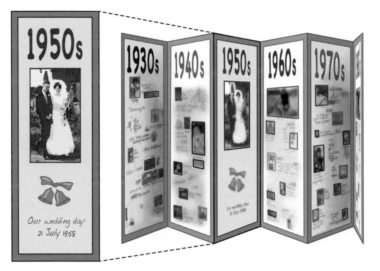

Figure 3.4a: Timeline using a paper-based column format

1930s	1940s	1950s	1960s	1970s	1980s	19
My parents met and married. Me born. Harry born.	Moved to Liverpool. Went to school. Met best friend, Vera.	Started work. Met John at a dance. Married John.	Alice was born. James was born.	Moved to Yorkshire. Went to France on holiday.	James graduated from university. Alice got married. First grandchild born.	

Figure 3.4b: Timeline using an online column format

The format of the timeline could also be a clock face. It could be split into decades, with entries in each sector.

Other information about a person's life

A biography or life history is not only about key life events. If you are to understand someone as they are now, you need to be appreciate much more about their life.

You should also find out about things such as:

* likes and dislikes
* beliefs and values
* habits and routines, e.g. getting the same train to work every day
* people, e.g. their partner, children, friends, colleagues
* animals, e.g. previous pets
* interests, e.g. gardening, cars, art, music
* achievements, e.g. promotions, awards, qualifications
* disappointments, e.g. failures, redundancy
* dreams and hopes
* sense of humour
* favourite places.

The benefits of putting together a life history

Biographies can be put together in a range of ways, such as in an album, on a chart, or on a computer. How they are done does not matter: the insights that you will gain into someone's life are the important results of doing this work.

Putting together a life history also provides the person with a useful tool to help recall their own history. For example, being able to look at a photograph can often help with orientation. Someone who is distressed because she 'has to get home to cook tea for her children' can be gently shown photographs of her children as adults, and encouraged to reorientate and refocus her thoughts.

Activity

Do this activity with a partner if you can. If not, make notes at each stage:

* Think about the information you would want to get across to others so that they could understand you.
* Look at the bullet points above listing other information about a person's life, such as likes and dislikes. Which of those factors, or other factors, would really help people to know about you?
* Tell your partner, or make notes, about all the important things people should know about your life.
* If you are working with a partner, swap roles and listen to what they have to say about their life.
* Now explain what you have been told, or noted down, to someone else, or to a group.

Knowing a person's history makes a huge difference to how you relate to them. If you are aware of a person's background it can help you to understand some of their behaviour. It is often possible to work out what someone is trying to communicate if you can think about what you know of their history.

Case study

Maria has dementia and she lives in a residential care home. She has been there for several years, and during that time her dementia has progressed. Staff at the home are finding it increasingly difficult to manage her behaviour. At mealtimes, Maria wanders around the dining room. She leans over other residents while they are eating and often grabs their knives or forks. Many of the residents do not have dementia and are complaining about her behaviour: some are quite upset and others are aggressive and angry. There have been serious discussions about having to move Maria to a nursing home or specialist facility.

When a life history was being prepared for Maria, it was discovered that she had been a children's nanny. She had literally 'mothered' dozens of different children throughout her life. It became clear that her behaviour was related to helping children to eat properly.

Once staff became aware of this, it was easier to manage her behaviour. A member of staff diverted her attention when she began to approach people at the table, reassuring her that everyone was eating properly and that she could sit down and enjoy her own meal.

1 How did knowing about Maria's life history change the understanding of her behaviour?
2 What might have happened if this information had not been discovered?

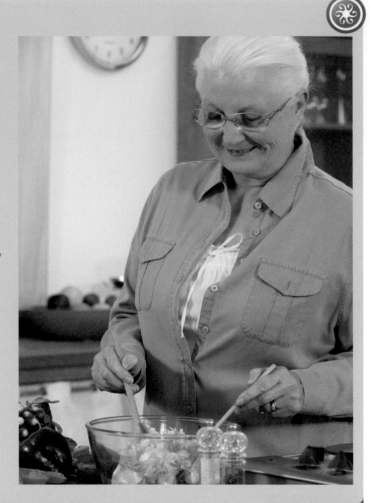

AC 205:3.2 and 210:2.1

3.2 Techniques that help to facilitate positive interactions

Practical techniques

Christine Bryden (née Boden) is an Australian woman with dementia. She has written a powerful book called *Who Will I Be When I Die?*

Christine was 46 when she was diagnosed with fronto-temporal lobe dementia. These are her suggestions for supporting communication with people who have dementia:

- **Give us time to speak**. Wait for us to search around that untidy heap on the floor of the brain for the word we want to use. Try not to finish our sentences. Just listen, and don't let us feel embarrassed if we lose the thread of what we say.

- **Don't rush us into something because we can't think or speak fast enough to let you know whether we agree**. Try to give us time to respond and to let you know whether we really want to do it.

- **When you want to talk to us, think of some way to do this without questions, which can alarm us or make us feel uncomfortable**. If we have forgotten something special that happened recently, don't assume it wasn't special for us too. Just give us a gentle prompt – we may just be momentarily blank.

- **Don't try too hard to help us remember something that just happened**. If it never registered, we are never going to be able to recall it.

- **Avoid background noise if you can**. If the TV is on, mute it first.

- **If children are underfoot, remember we will get tired very easily and find it very hard to concentrate on talking and listening as well**. Maybe one child at a time and without background noise would be best.

- **Earplugs** may be useful if visiting shopping centres or other noisy places.

Positive person work

The Bradford Dementia Group, led by Professor Tom Kitwood, developed a set of key aspects of positive interactions that Kitwood called positive person work.

This work is part of the person-centred approach to dementia care and is used in a process of 'mapping' dementia care in order to better understand the world in which each individual lives. The work identifies 17 'personal enhancers' that support positive interactions, promote the 'personhood' of the person with dementia, and improve and enhance lives. These enhancers should ensure a positive atmosphere in a residential setting, and support people with dementia to focus on their strengths and make the most of their abilities.

This approach will be explored in more detail in a later chapter. As a taster, the enhancers include:

- **warmth** – showing real care, interest and concern for people
- **holding** – offering safety and security so that people can be reassured and feel comforted
- **celebration** – valuing and recognising people's achievements
- **genuineness** – being truthful, clear and honest
- **empowerment** – putting people in control of their own lives; letting go of the power of the professional
- **belonging** – making sure people feel accepted and part of the community in which they are living
- **fun** – enjoying humour and sharing laughter with people; encouraging people to look at the lighter side.

Activity

Look at each of the enhancers in the bullet points above.

Make some notes about how each enhancer could make a difference to your interactions with people with dementia. Be clear about how each enhancer could make interactions more positive.

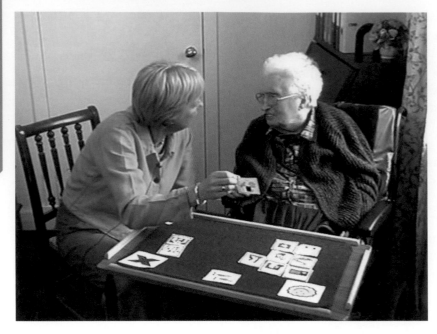

Talking mats® can help people with dementia engage in a positive interaction.

The Bradford technique of interpreting, exploring and repairing is relevant to these outcomes because it advocates life history in interpreting and exploring. It also provides suggestions for 'repairing' conversations, stating that the value of communication is sometimes more important than the content.

More than words

For some people, words are not enough and pictures can often be the best way of conducting a positive interaction. The University of Stirling have developed Talking Mats® that help people to use clear and simple symbols to communicate.

Simple cards can also be handmade quite easily, as long as people are clear about what the symbols mean and that everyone who is going to use them understands how they work.

Doing it well

Being prepared to think about the right communication methods is one effective way of showing a commitment to person-centred working.

Here is a checklist of practical techniques you can use to facilitate positive interactions:

- Show that you are giving your full attention.
- Reduce or stop background noise.
- Speak clearly in a steady, calm way.
- Use simple, short sentences.
- Be prepared to wait for a response.
- Do not finish someone's sentences.
- Listen carefully.
- Observe and respond to body language.
- Be aware of your body language.
- Use touch to reassure and communicate.
- Gently divert conversation away from confused ideas – do not challenge or argue.
- Use pictures or written communication, where appropriate.
- Remember to consider that someone might be in pain, or have a physical condition that may affect interaction.
- Check glasses, hearing aids and dentures.
- Show genuine respect and care for the person.
- Find out about people's life and history – you will be surprised at how much they have done.

3.3 How involving others can enhance interaction

AC 205:3.3

Plenty of other people are likely to be involved in the care and support of each person with dementia that you are supporting. Some of them will be informal family and friend carers. There will also be other professionals supporting the person in some part of their life.

Other professionals could include (as mentioned in the previous chapter):

- social worker
- occupational therapist
- speech and language therapist
- pharmacist
- physiotherapist
- nurse
- dementia care advisor
- GP
- psychologist
- psychiatrist
- advocate.

Sometimes involving another person can help interactions. They might have a greater knowledge of the person than you do, or have a particularly good relationship with them so that the person is more likely to trust and be relaxed with them.

Alternatively, other professionals may have valuable information to share:

- A **speech and language therapist** may be able to suggest ways to address some communication issues.
- A **pharmacist** or **GP** may be able to advise how the side effects of medication might impact on how well a person can communicate.
- A **social worker** may be able to provide useful information about a person's history and family situation, which may help to explain particular behaviours or attitudes.
- The **dementia care advisor** is likely to be able to offer advice and direct you to useful guidance to improve interactions.
- An **advocate** will be able to offer a view from the perspective of the person with dementia, to provide information about the person's capacity and what is considered to be in their best interests.

Not everyone will have all of these professionals involved in supporting them. However, if possible it is valuable to involve them so that they can contribute towards positive and useful interactions and relationships.

Family and friends may also be able to support positive contact with someone with dementia. Again, they will have information and advice about the best methods of communication, and they may help increase the person's confidence.

Always consider if there is something to be gained by involving another person. Potential sources of assistance in improving and promoting good conversation and relationships are to be welcomed and used to full advantage. That way you can be sure that you have done everything possible to put the person with dementia at the centre of your practice.

Getting ready for assessment

DEM 205 is a knowledge-based unit. You will be asked to show that you have understood each of the three learning outcomes. This unit does not require the demonstration of skills, so does not have to be assessed in the workplace. You may have to prepare an assignment or a presentation, or you could be asked to answer a series of questions, possibly in a professional discussion with your assessor.

Even though this unit does not assess skills, you should try to relate your learning to the workplace wherever possible. Use anonymised examples of people you support to illustrate your points, and refer to the communication practices of your own workplace wherever possible.

Relating the knowledge to your own practice will help to show your assessor that you have understood what you have learned and are going to be able to put it into practice.

DEM 210 is a competence-based unit and requires that you demonstrate your skills in the workplace. You will need to be able to show your assessor that you are able to communicate and interact effectively with people with dementia.

Your assessor will also want you to demonstrate that you work in a person-centred way and put the person at the centre of all your practice. You will need to ensure that you have understood the reasons why you are working in this way, and why certain approaches, attitudes and behaviours are likely to result in the best outcomes for people with dementia.

Further reading and research

- Dementia Gateway has a large number of resources that support working with people who have dementia, including case studies. See the Social Care Institute for Excellence website at www.scie.org.uk for more information.

- The Alzheimer's Society website has plenty of information on communicating with people who have dementia: see www.alzheimers.org.uk.

- There are some useful resources on the Dementia Positive website, as a result of the work of John Killick and Kate Allan. For more information on how to approach dementia in a positive and constructive way, see www.dementiapositive.co.uk.

- The Princess Royal Trust for Carers website includes resources that focus on family carers for people who have dementia: see www.carers.org.

Chapter 4:
Equality, diversity and inclusion in dementia care

Ensuring that people are treated equally and fairly, and are not discriminated against, is important for anyone who uses services.

People with dementia are among the most vulnerable, and their interests need to be protected. The nature of dementia and its progress can mean that people are not always aware of discrimination or of being excluded. Many people find it hard to know how to include someone with dementia and so it is easier not to think about them and to ignore them. People do not always understand the needs that a person with dementia has, and how to make sure that they are included in all aspects of life.

Learners who have studied unit SHC 23 may find some of this material familiar, as the principles of acknowledging diversity, equality and inclusion are the same, whichever group you support.

When you have achieved these units you will:

- understand the importance of equality, diversity and inclusion when working with people with dementia
- understand and be able to apply a person-centred approach when supporting people with dementia
- understand and be able to work with a range of people who have dementia to ensure that diverse needs are met.

> **Key term**
>
> **Diversity** – relates to difference and the richness and variety that different people bring to society.

1: The importance of equality, diversity and inclusion

1.1 What do diversity, equality and inclusion mean?

Diversity

Diversity is about difference. The value of diversity is the richness and variety that different people bring to society.

The statement that 'all cars are silver' is clearly silly. Of course they're not – cars can be any colour.

When it comes to people, everyone is different. There are many ways in which people differ from each other, including:

- appearance
- gender
- race
- culture
- ability
- talents
- beliefs.

The importance of diversity

Imagine how boring life would be if everyone was exactly the same. Whole societies of identical 'cloned' people have been the central theme of films: it is clear immediately how unnatural it is. However, we are not always very good at recognising and valuing the differences in the people we meet.

When working in a person-centred way with people with dementia, a vitally important activity is to find out about their life history in detail, so that you can understand the *whole* person and see how their personal history has contributed to making them who they are. This 'biography' will also tell you all the special and unique things about them and the individual contributions they have made during their lifetime. Recognising and valuing all of this is part of what diversity is about.

You can think about diversity in two main ways:

1 There are *specific* differences between people: all of the features that make each of us an individual.

2 There are *broader* differences between people, as you can see from the bullet points above.

Both of these are important. You need to take account of each of them, and value the contributions that are made by different perspectives, different ways of thinking and different approaches.

Activity

This exercise is best done with a group of colleagues, but you can also do it on your own.

- Write down all the cultures and nationalities you can think of as a list.
- Next to each one, write something that the culture has given to the world. For example, the Arab culture gave us mathematics, the Chinese have developed some wonderful medicines, etc.
- Next, think about the different people you support. Note down the special angle of understanding each person can bring to society. For instance, someone who is visually impaired will judge people on how they behave, not on how they look. Older people can often bring a different perspective to a situation, based on years of experience and understanding. Someone who remembers less than they used to and struggles with words may communicate using touch and gestures, a very gentle and special way to make contact with someone.
- Make notes on each of the ideas you come up with.

You may find it helpful to do some research in the light of this activity: you may find some fascinating information in the process.

Reflect

When you have completed the activity, be honest with yourself about whether you have really appreciated and valued the differences in individuals and cultures in the past.

How do you think that valuing the importance of diversity could improve your practice?

Equality

How can you foster and encourage **equality**, which seems to be about everyone being equal, alongside diversity, which is about everyone being different? It is not as impossible as it appears.

The key concept to understand is that what you are being asked to do is to promote 'equality' – which is not necessarily the same thing as treating everyone the same.

Confused?

Think about a running race. Everyone would agree that, generally, for a race to be fair, all the competitors must be on the start line and start at the same time.

Before people have a chance to take part in the race, they have to reach the start line. Yet many people in our society need considerable help just to reach the 'start line' before they can even begin to 'take part in the race'. If you are to support people in reaching the start line, you have to be able to find out from them what additional support they are going to need.

Key term

Equality – treating people equally: it is not the same thing as treating everyone the same.

Case studies

Elizabeth

Elizabeth is in her late 70s, but is very fit and active. She was a head teacher until she retired over 15 years ago. Since then, she has travelled all over the world, and is very involved in a local history group and with her local community council.

She began to become forgetful and realised that she was having more trouble than other friends of her age in remembering words, and having sufficient concentration to read her morning paper and remember what she had read.

Elizabeth was diagnosed as having the early stages of dementia. Once she had begun to come to terms with the diagnosis, she researched all she could find out about dementia and the opportunities available. She organised and recruited friends for support as needed, but wanted to have some professional involvement as a back-up.

Ed

Ed is 67. He was diagnosed with Alzheimer's disease a couple of years ago after his wife died. His condition had been deteriorating for some years, but his wife had covered up for his

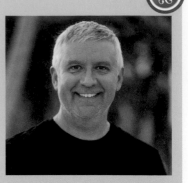

increasing forgetfulness, mood swings and confusion, and it had not really been obvious to his family until she died suddenly.

Initially, his family put his depression and withdrawn state down to grief after losing his wife, but it became clear that he was not coping. Both his children lived far away and neither was able to visit more frequently than every other weekend. Ed had been picked up by the police on a few occasions as he was lost and saying he needed to get to work – he had been employed in a local factory all his working life. Neighbours would also bring him back and he regularly went out leaving his front door wide open.

On the last occasion when the police brought him back, they found the gas turned on and the front door open. They contacted Social Services as they were concerned about the risk that Ed was presenting to himself, and possibly to his neighbours.

Can you see why Elizabeth and Ed needed entirely different levels of support, even though they both had dementia, and how what worked for one would not have worked for the other?

Treating these two people the same would not have resulted in equality. The equality comes from the fact that both of them had their needs met. Elizabeth would have hated a setting where she was looked after and supported 24 hours a day. She was at a stage in her life where she wanted to manage in her own way for as long as possible. Conversely, Ed would have been lost if given only a little back-up support.

You are most likely to hear about equality in relation to 'equality of opportunity': this is about everyone having the same chances to live a safe, healthy, happy and productive life.

Inclusion

Inclusion is, as it sounds, about making sure that people are included and not left out. Supporting people to take part in society is supporting inclusion. Often, ensuring that people are included is about moving barriers that are in the way and that are stopping people from taking part.

Barriers to inclusion

The different sorts of barriers to inclusion include:

- **physical barriers**, such as access
- **intellectual barriers**, where people are excluded because they cannot respond or participate quickly as a result of conditions such as dementia

- **language barriers** – either speaking a different language, or using jargon that people cannot understand
- **financial barriers** – where cost can mean that some people cannot take part
- **emotional barriers**, because people feel intimidated or they lack confidence
- **lack of information** – people may not realise that certain things are available, or know how to access them.

You can see how people with dementia can be excluded from day-to-day life because they may communicate in a different way than people expect, or they may not always be clear about where they are in time and place. It is difficult to participate in many activities if you are not always sure how to make sense of the words you are reading, the numbers on a bus, or if you get confused making choices about what meal you want to eat.

Inclusive practice

Definitions of inclusive practice are varied, but broadly it is about ensuring that there are no barriers that would exclude or make it difficult for people to participate fully in society. People must be included in all aspects of life, not excluded from some of them because of an illness or a disability.

Traditionally, we have developed separate worlds in order to meet people's needs. Examples include separate workshops, education groups and living accommodation for people with mental health needs, dementia or other types of disability. These types of arrangements have kept a range of people out of the mainstream of society.

Older people have had separate clubs, day centres and residential accommodation on the assumption that 'separate is best'. Increasingly, we have come to see that *separate is not equal*, and we should have an inclusive society that everyone can enjoy.

Now we are asking different questions about how we organise society:

- We are not asking, 'What is wrong with this person that means they cannot use the leisure centre or the cinema?'
- Instead, we are asking, 'What is wrong with the cinema or the leisure centre if people with disabilities can't use it?'

Inclusive practice is about providing the support that people want in order to live their lives as fully as possible.

Examples of inclusive practice are:

- changing the physical shape and colour of buildings to reduce confusion for people with dementia
- providing plenty of spaces where people with dementia can walk or pace if they want to
- having large, clear signs to provide information
- ensuring that systems and processes for obtaining support are easy to use, with clear, simple choices and support if needed.

Overall, practising in an inclusive way means constantly asking about the changes that need to happen so that a person can participate, and then doing whatever is within our area of responsibility to make those changes happen. In order to make it possible for anyone to be included in society, we all have to make the necessary changes happen.

1.2 Unique needs and preferences of people with dementia

Everyone has unique and individual needs, as you saw in the case study about Elizabeth and Ed in the previous section.

Two people can have the same condition but very different needs, and make very different choices about how to manage their lives. The whole point of a person-centred approach is to ensure that people are able to make the choices that express their own needs and preferences. A person with dementia is no different from any other person who has support from professional carers: they need to be in control of their own lives, and the support they receive must be to meet *their* needs and not the needs of the service.

Although everyone with dementia is an individual with their own needs, there are some general issues that are common to most people with dementia. One of the biggest issues that people face is the general lack of understanding about dementia amongst society as a whole. There is an assumption that people with dementia are incapable of looking after themselves, making any decisions or running their own lives. Nothing could be further from the truth, certainly in the early stages of dementia. It is important that there is a greater awareness of what dementia really means and how people can be supported.

Local communities

People with dementia need local communities to support them. The attitude and involvement of friends, neighbours and the local community can make a huge difference to whether people are able to retain their independence and stay in their own homes. More than for many other conditions, the level of support can make a major difference to how dementia impacts on people's lives as it progresses.

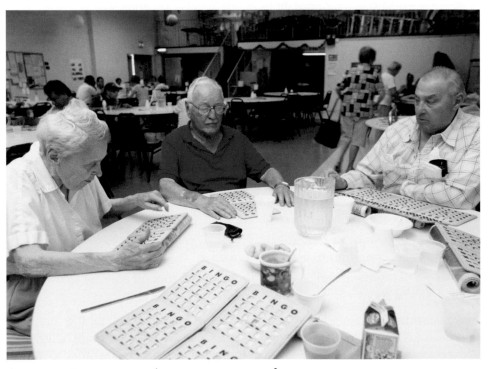

A community centre can be a great source of support.

Local communities can help in a range of ways, for instance:

- neighbours can keep an eye on the person and be aware of potential 'warning' signs: an open door, milk on the step, etc.
- local shops can keep a list of essential shopping items, so that important items are not forgotten
- local pharmacies can support people with medication.

All of these actions can help people to keep on making their own choices about their lives.

Activity

Think of a person you support and make a list of the needs they have (regardless of whether or not these are currently being met).

Now think about the needs they will have in the foreseeable future.

Make a list of how needs are being – and could be – met now, and how needs could be met in the future.

Supporting carers

Many carers have been undertaking their caring role for a long time and are used to meeting the needs of their loved one. However, sometimes this closeness can mean that needs are not always recognised or preferences acted upon. You will often hear, 'We always do it like this', or 'He prefers it this way', or 'She doesn't like to…'. This is not because people are unthinking, but because caring for someone with dementia is very demanding. Continuing to do things as they have always been done may seem the easier way, rather than risking trying anything new.

Working closely with carers so that they are able to recognise the value of person-centred working is important, and can be rewarding. Often, carers will be amazed and delighted at the change in the person they love, as they understand how to meet individual needs by responding to behaviour as a means of communication rather than as a symptom of the dementia.

Being a carer can be a very lonely life. When carers are introduced to the idea of support being provided by the local community, it can take a huge load from their shoulders and they may welcome involvement from others. Similarly, carers often think that they should take on all the caring responsibilities themselves and are reluctant to ask for help. Finding that there are other people willing to offer support can be a great relief.

It is not always easy for carers to reach the view that there may be another way of doing things, especially if they have been caring for a person for a long time. Always show people person-centred approaches in action, perhaps by agreeing a visit to a local facility where it is operating. It is always easier to show people something in practice rather than just try to explain it. It is also important to take the time to explain how an approach works in the context of their loved one. If you are supporting the person, you can demonstrate through your own approach the difference it can make when a person's unique needs are recognised and responded to.

Doing it well

Here are some reminders about what to remember when you are supporting carers:

- Be sensitive to people's feelings.
- Value the work that the carers are doing.
- Explain and give information in a way that people can use.
- Reinforce verbal information with written details.
- Show people how the approach works in action if they wish.
- Use your own work as an example.

Everyone likes to receive information in a way that suits them:

- Some people welcome written information about the way you are working.
- Others prefer a verbal discussion and the opportunity to look through written information later.

If you have the task of explaining person-centred approaches to a carer, make sure that you find out the best way to give them information. Use your communication skills to give information in a way that does not appear to criticise how they are currently caring for their loved one with dementia. Be sensitive to how some people may respond if they feel that they are not being valued and appreciated.

AC 207:1.3 and 209:1.5

Above all, make sure that carers can see the possible benefits for all concerned of putting the person with dementia in control of their life: in control of making sure that their needs are known and that everyone understands their preferences about how to meet them.

1.3 Values, beliefs and misunderstandings about dementia

Cultural attitudes

Western cultures

In Western cultures we do not generally value old age: we tend to view older people as needing assistance, being decrepit and not able to make a useful contribution to society. There is little respect or recognition of the contribution that older people have made, or are still able to make.

Even where there is a caring attitude to older people, it can be patronising and assume that they need to be looked after. It is not unusual for older people to be treated as if they are children and spoken to in a 'sing song' voice, addressed by their first name without asking permission to do so, and to have their hands patted as if they are a child in need of comfort.

Eastern cultures

The approach to old age is different in many other cultures, particularly in many Eastern countries. Older people are valued for their wisdom: they are seen as important and as having an important place in both the family and society in general.

Signs of change

There are some signs of change in Western societies. As people over the age of 60 make up larger proportions of the population, it has become clear that there are not enough young people in the workforce to support the number of retired people, so many companies are recruiting older people. The Equality Act has made it illegal to discriminate against people on the grounds of age, so more older people are remaining an active part of the workforce.

Changes in attitudes, however, will take many years to come about. In the meantime, older people can be dismissed, ridiculed or patronised.

False beliefs and misunderstandings about dementia

Although not everyone with dementia is an older person, the vast majority are. Out of the approximately 750,000 people with dementia in the UK, there are around 16,000 who are under 65, and so the attitudes to dementia are bound up with attitudes towards ageing.

There is a **stigma** associated with dementia that makes it difficult for people to talk about, or to be willing to recognise the signs. A study by the Alzheimer's Society in 2002, *Feeling the Pulse*, found that people currently wait up to three years before reporting symptoms to their doctor.

This applies not only to individuals and their families, but also to professionals: they are not always quick to recognise the symptoms of dementia and will often tell people that memory loss is 'just a sign of old age'.

There is also a completely false idea among both the public and professionals that there is nothing that can be done about dementia, so there is little point in looking at any treatment or support systems.

The *Facing Dementia Survey* (Eisai, Inc and Pfizer, Inc, 2004) stated that:

- 70 per cent of carers report being unaware of the symptoms of dementia before diagnosis
- 64 per cent of carers report being in denial about their relative having the illness
- 58 per cent of carers believe the symptoms to be just part of ageing
- 50 per cent of the public believe that there is a stigma attached to dementia.

Living Well with Dementia, the government's national dementia strategy, suggests that public and professional knowledge and attitudes are a barrier to the diagnosis of dementia and the provision of good-quality care and support.

> **Key term**
>
> **Stigma** – a mark of disgrace associated with a particular circumstance, quality or person.

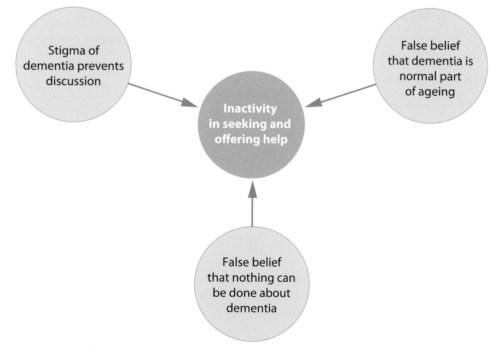

Figure 4.1: The impact of the stigma and false beliefs surrounding dementia

Lack of awareness

It seems that a combination of our society's attitudes to ageing and a great deal of ignorance and lack of understanding about dementia contribute to the fear and stigma associated with it. If people were more aware that dementia can be treated and improved, perhaps there would be less reluctance to seek help in the early stages.

One of the problems caused by the lack of awareness of the true facts about dementia is that people assume that the symptoms are just part of growing old and that there is nothing that can be done. It is true that dementia cannot be cured. However, there is much that can be done to slow its progress, to treat it and to improve people's health and well-being while they live with the condition. If there was more understanding of the importance of seeking help early, then more people would be able to plan effective ways of living well with dementia.

Activity

Try carrying out your own informal survey about people's attitudes and understanding of dementia. Ask friends and family, any carers of people you support, and any other professionals with whom you come into contact.

You can make your survey very informal because it is just to find out about people's attitudes. If you find it helpful, try asking the following questions:

1   Do you think that dementia is a normal part of ageing?
2   Can anything be done about dementia?
3   What do you think a GP can offer someone with dementia?
4   Name three sources of help for people with dementia or their families.

Changing attitudes: key messages about dementia

The government's dementia strategy identifies some key messages that need to be made clear to the general public:

- Dementia is a condition.
- Dementia is common.
- Dementia is not an inevitable consequence of ageing.
- The social environment is important, and quality of life is as related to the richness of interactions and relationships as it is to the extent of brain disease.
- Dementia is not an immediate death sentence: there is life to be lived with dementia and it can be of good quality.
- There is an immense number of positive things that we can do – as family members, friends and professionals – to improve the quality of life of people with dementia.
- People with dementia make, and can continue to make, a positive contribution to their communities. Most of us will experience some form of dementia either ourselves or through someone we care about.
- We can all play a part in protecting and supporting people with dementia and their carers.
- Our risk of dementia may be reduced if we protect our general health, e.g. by eating a healthy diet, stopping smoking, exercising regularly, drinking less alcohol and generally protecting the brain from injury.

2: Understanding and applying a person-centred approach

2.1 How people with dementia can feel valued and included

■ Learning outcomes
207:2, 209:1 and 209:2

AC 207:2.1

Valuing people as *individuals* is a key part of a person-centred approach.

Bradford University has developed much of the work around person-centred approaches to dementia. One framework they work with is called VIPS:

- **V**aluing – unconditional valuing of the person with dementia, their carers and the professional staff. This is about valuing everyone, and recognising that person-centred approaches are about everyone involved, not just the person with dementia.

- **I**ndividualised – recognising and responding to the person as a unique individual.

- **P**erspective – seeing the world from the person's viewpoint.

- **S**upportive – making sure that the person's environment is positive and supports their well-being.

It is easy to forget the factors that may make people with dementia feel that they do not belong, or that they cannot participate in what is going on around them.

It can be simple things such as:

- people talking too quickly, so that the person with dementia cannot process the information

- a person asking too many questions

- information being communicated in a format or style that the person with dementia cannot understand

- a situation involving lots of people that the person with dementia does not know

- being in a strange place.

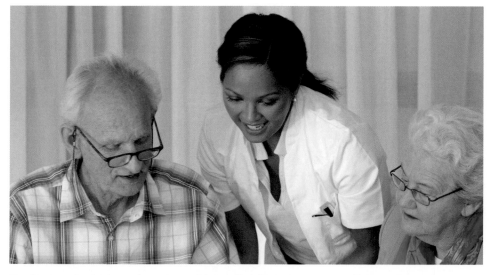

Feeling included can have great benefits for a person's self-esteem and self-confidence.

Other factors can be more complex and harder to resolve. Examples include:

- there being a complicated system to access services
- buildings being a confusing design
- the local community not being supportive
- the local area not being easy to walk around
- service providers changing staff frequently.

Although it may be easier to sort out the simpler factors, the more difficult issues do need to be addressed if people are going to feel that they are included and involved.

You may not be able to solve issues personally, but you do have a responsibility to report issues that are causing people to feel excluded, and to highlight them to your line manager(s) so that problems can be considered. There is a strong chance that attitudes that fail to value people or that fail to work in an inclusive way will result in discrimination against individuals, or against a whole group of people.

AC 207:2.2 and 209:1.3

2.2 How people with dementia may feel excluded

Discrimination

Discrimination is the result of behaviour that excludes, or fails to include, people. This can happen because of thoughtlessness or lack of care, but the basic cause comes from thinking in stereotypes.

Stereotyping is when we make assumptions that all people in one particular group are the same: stereotyping is an 'easy' way of thinking about the world. Stereotypes might suggest that all people over 65 are frail and walk with a stick, that all black young people who live in inner cities are on drugs, that all Muslims are terrorists, or that all families have a mother, father and two children. These stereotypes are often reinforced by the media or by advertising. Television programmes will often portray violent, criminal characters as young and black, and older people as being dependent and unable to make a useful contribution to society.

If you look back at the case studies in Section 1.1 on page 80, you can see that although Elizabeth and Ed both had dementia, they were very different, had led very different lives, and had completely different needs. If you had made an assumption that, because they both had dementia, their needs were the same, it is unlikely that either of them would have had their needs met.

The effect of stereotypes is to make you jump to conclusions about people. Have you ever felt uneasy seeing a young man with a shaved head walking towards you? You know nothing about him, but the way he looks makes you form an opinion about him. Do you have a picture in your mind of a social worker or a police officer? Think about how much the media influences that – do police officers and social workers all look like that?

The same principle applies to the stereotype of a person with dementia. There is an assumption that all people with dementia sit in chairs mumbling to themselves, or wander about getting lost. There is an assumption that they are completely unable to care for themselves or to have any kind of independence.

Key terms

Discrimination – the result of behaviour that excludes, or fails to include, people.

Stereotyping – making assumptions that all people in a particular group are the same.

This stereotype is as wrong as the assumption that all young people wearing a hooded top are muggers.

Professor Tom Kitwood, as part of his person-centred approach to dementia, identifies 'malignant social psychology'. This is where the attitudes and approach of professional staff will reduce the 'personhood' of someone. This can include:

- treating people like children
- devaluing what people can do
- assuming that someone with dementia can do nothing
- assuming that all people with dementia are the same and are having the same experience.

These attitudes are not intentionally abusive, but they can make people feel devalued, inhuman and no longer a person.

Reflect

Stop yourself every time you make a generalisation. Take a moment to look at the prejudice that is behind what you have said. Think about why you are thinking the way you do, and do something about it.

For example, next time you hear yourself saying, 'Social workers never understand what is really needed', 'GPs always take ages to visit' or 'People who live here wouldn't be interested in that', stop and think about what you are saying.

It may be true that some social workers will not understand – maybe all of those you have met so far! However, that does not necessarily apply to them all. Perhaps most of the people you support would not be interested in whatever was being suggested, but some might. You cannot make that assumption. You need to ask. People must be able to make choices because they are all different. Do not fall into the trap of stereotyping individuals based on factors such as gender, age, race, culture, dress or where they live.

Anti-discriminatory practice

In order to make sure that the people you support do not suffer discrimination, it is important that you practise in an anti-discriminatory way. **Anti-discriminatory practice** is what underpins good social care. For you to practise in a way that reduces discrimination, much of what you do in your day-to-day work with people with dementia must be based on anti-discriminatory practice. You need to think carefully about how people you support can be subject to discrimination because of the way that they are thought of by the general public.

Consider in your own workplace if activities and day-to-day living are organised without thinking about the *individuals* involved. Is there an assumption that everyone will want to do the same things simply because they all have dementia?

Your day-to-day practice and attitudes have a strong bearing on how effective your anti-discriminatory practice will be. There is little point in supporting someone to challenge stereotyping and then returning to your own work setting to organise all the 'ladies' for a sewing afternoon!

Key term

Anti-discriminatory practice – working in ways that challenge discrimination.

Activity

Think of three examples of discrimination: the examples can be from work, from other parts of your life or from fiction.

For each example, look at how you could work in a way that is anti-discriminatory in order to reduce the effect of the discrimination.

AC 209:2.1

2.3 Taking life history into consideration to meet needs

The importance of someone's life history

Someone's history is what makes them the person they are now. Just because they have dementia does not mean that they are not still an individual with their own special story about their life, their likes and dislikes, hopes, fears and dreams like everyone else. This topic is also covered in Chapter 3.

A life history is more than just about recording a series of life events. Life events are important, but more needs to be included in order to get a full picture of the individual – everything that is important in the person's life.

A life history should include:

- beliefs and values
- likes and dislikes – not just dietary likes and dislikes, but in all aspects of life
- important life events, accomplishments, achievements and disappointments
- people who are important, e.g. partner, family, friends, neighbours, colleagues
- pets – current and previous
- important places and belongings
- the person's skills and talents
- interests and any hobbies – current or previous
- education and work life
- habits, and how the person likes to behave
- what makes them happy or sad
- what they find funny.

Life histories are very useful in helping to make sure that people have their needs met in the best possible way. If you know about a person's background and history, it may help you to understand their present behaviour, or to find out about routines that could be useful. Life histories can also help with explaining some of the words or expressions that people may use. Phrases or sayings that are familiar to members of their family may seem odd if you do not know the person. Having the information will help your understanding and improve your ability to communicate well with the person.

If you know about a person's strengths and some of the hardships or great achievements of their lives, it can help you to understand what they are likely to be able to do for themselves, e.g. how an apparently frail person is actually very tough and strong emotionally, and may have survived and overcome great hardships.

Overall, recording a person's life history can help you to get to know someone and to feel more involved with them and their lives. It all helps you to see the *person* and *not* the dementia. Life histories can also be useful for younger family members who may have no idea of the life their older relative has led: looking at a life history can help them to see the real person and understand that there has been much more to the person than they see now.

The process of gathering a life history is also a useful one. For many people, the opportunity to talk about their lives is enjoyable, and recalling memories and telling you about their past is really beneficial. Do not make the sessions too much like hard work: short sessions over a period of time is better than making people sit for hours. Depending on the stage of the dementia, sessions of about five minutes may be all that a person can manage. Others may be happy to talk to you for half an hour or more.

How to record a life history

There is no set way of gathering and recording a life history:

1 You could use a standard template if your organisation has one. There are some advantages to this as it means that you know where to look for specific pieces of information.

2 You could use an album style where there is a mix of information, stories, photographs and letters or cards that are important to the person. This can be something that people will enjoy looking through and talking about.

For some people, and particularly as the generation who use social networking grow older, life histories can be gathered and recorded using mobile technology. This develops the idea much further, because video, music and very large numbers of photographs can be used and easily accessed on devices such as iPads.

Case study

Jack has late-stage dementia. He is very disorientated, but is comforted by having his hand held and looking through books on local history with lots of photographs.

The major difficulty for Jack is that he becomes very agitated and distressed just before breakfast each morning: he begins shouting and trying to get out of the home. Staff have been spending a fair bit of time trying to calm him down and get him to come and sit down for breakfast. They have done their best to work out why breakfast is so upsetting for him and have tried various options, such as serving him in his room and serving him in the lounge, but nothing seems to help him.

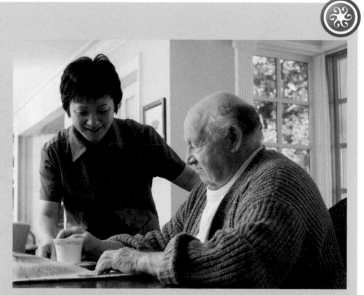

In the process of putting together Jack's life history, one of his daughters happens to say that he worked in the same office for 50 years and caught the 7.30am train every morning like clockwork. She said that he always left at exactly the same time and was a man who was very orderly and followed strict routines.

just for a short walk. Once he had his walk, Jack would then happily come in and eat breakfast.

Knowing Jack's life history made it much easier to realise the cause of his distress. It was included into Jack's support plan that every morning someone would go out into the garden with him,

1 How did the morning walk help Jack?

2 What may have happened if Jack's life history had not been gathered?

AC 207:2.3

2.4 Including people in all aspects of their care

Social care has moved on from the days when we did things *to* people and provided people with whatever we, as professionals, considered to be best for them. Over the last few years, we have come to understand that people are still in control of their lives. Needing support from social care professionals does not mean that a person has to give up choice and control over their life.

It is important that people are involved in all aspects of their lives and are not just passive receivers of 'care'. This is not just about deciding on support packages. It is also about making sure that people have a real input into what happens to them on a day-to-day basis: from choosing clothes to self-medication. It is also about issues such as deciding when and where to go out, when to get up and go to bed, and how to spend free time.

An individual's ability to be involved in all the different aspects of their support will vary depending on the stage and nature of their dementia. However, the opportunity should always be there and nothing should be done without offering the person the opportunity to state their views. For some people their ability to be involved will vary, as their condition may be changeable. It may be that someone in the early stages of dementia will be able to state their wishes very clearly and enter into discussions around some of the bigger issues. A person in the later stages may find that difficult, but may still be able to understand and communicate using various techniques including flash cards, simple questions, pictures and touch.

Working in this way when people have dementia does have risks, and these must be taken into account. For example, everyone should be encouraged to self-medicate, but all the risks have to be considered. Someone in the early stages of dementia can be supported to manage their own medication for as long as possible. Clearly, someone who is in the later stages and who is very disorientated, with serious memory loss, would not be able to take responsibility for their own medication. However, this does not mean that they should not be involved as far

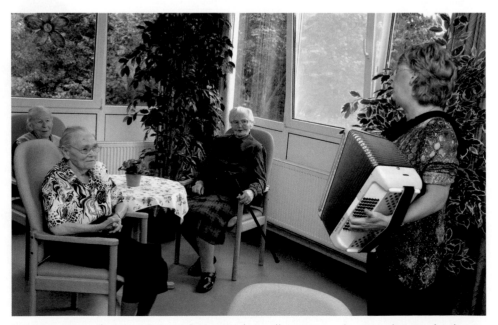

It is important that you learn what people really want to do on a day-to-day basis.

as possible, even if it is simply to physically take their own medication rather than have it put in their mouth by someone else.

As you work with someone with dementia, you will become quite skilled at communicating with them, so it will be possible for you to seek their views and wishes about day-to-day aspects of their life. Questions will need to be straightforward and only require a simple answer. The information that you know about the person from their life history will also help. For example, if you know someone has been a keen gardener and you are seeing how they would like to spend the afternoon, you could try asking, 'Would you like to come and sit in the garden?' For someone in the later stages of dementia, do not ask, 'What would you like to do this afternoon?' The question is too 'open' and complex, and will be very hard to process for the person.

The support that people have selected in order to help them to live well with their dementia is not only about day-to-day living and personal care. There are bigger issues such as how people relate to their local community, which family and friends they want to see regularly, and how a person wants to socialise with others. There are also important discussions around medicines, treatment and how people wish to experience the end of their life. These elements of support should be discussed and the person's wishes recorded as early as possible in the course of their dementia, so that you can be sure that you are able to find out their wishes.

3: Meeting a diverse range of individual needs

3.1 Different experiences of older and younger people

■ **Learning outcome**
207:3 and 209:3

AC 207:3.1 and 209:3.2

People with dementia share many similarities, but equally, there are a significant number of differences based on a range of different circumstances and backgrounds.

Age

One of the major differences is the age at which dementia begins. The majority of people with dementia are over the age of 65, but there are considerable numbers of younger people, mainly between the ages of 50 and 65, who have conditions that cause dementia. The Dementia UK Report (2007) estimates that there are around 18,000 younger people with dementia in the UK. This represents about 2 per cent of people with dementia and about 6 per cent of people from black and minority ethnic communities who have dementia.

It is difficult to be precise about the age at which dementia can begin, because older people are less likely to have a diagnosis in the early stages: memory loss and mild confusion are assumed to be part of growing older and are often ignored by people and unrecognised by health professionals. People under the age of 65 who develop symptoms are more likely to seek diagnosis because they do not expect to experience those types of symptoms at their age.

The most frequent form of dementia seen in younger people is fronto-temporal dementia. However, many people also develop Alzheimer's disease and vascular dementia while they are under the age of 65. Alcohol-related dementia –

Korsakoff's syndrome – is more common in younger people, as is Creutzfeld-Jakob disease and HIV-related dementia. For more information on different forms of dementia, see Chapter 1.

The conditions that cause dementia may be the same for all ages, but the impact of dementia on younger people can be very different from its impact on older people, which can result in some quite different needs.

Diagnosis

It can be difficult to diagnose most forms of dementia in younger people.

- Early onset dementia is not common, so most GPs have little experience in diagnosing it. The early stages of dementia are often mistaken for depression, menopause or substance abuse.
- Younger people with dementia can often have a problem in getting specialist treatment, as the medical specialities (e.g. older people's mental health, geriatric medicine) with the expertise are usually designed for older people.
- Early diagnosis is very important, as younger people with dementia are likely to have more commitments and need to be involved in long-term planning as soon as possible.

Personal and family life

If people with dementia have a dependent family, they need to think about what plans to make for the future.

- Younger people with dementia are more likely to have younger children, who may find it very hard to accept or understand the personality changes that result from dementia. These personality changes can cause real challenges for families.
- Young children lose the support of at least one parent, but often both, as one takes on the role of carer.
- Parents of younger people with dementia may be unwilling to accept the diagnosis, finding it hard to understand how it is possible that it is their child – and not them – who has dementia.

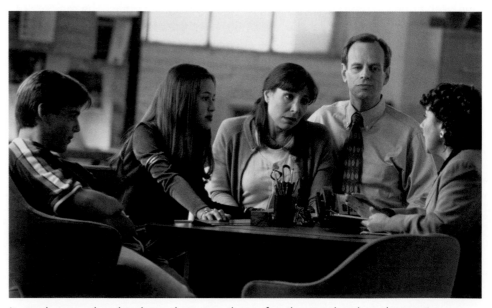

It can be very hard to hear the news that a family member has dementia.

- Friends and relatives may have difficulty accepting the diagnosis, and there may be less support available.
- Young people with dementia may experience changes in their sex lives: either a reduction or loss of interest in sex, or increased sexual demands, both of which may cause relationship problems.

Behaviour

There is a lack of awareness among the public of early onset dementia, so behaviours associated with dementia may not be tolerated in the same way as they would with an older person:

- Younger people with dementia are more likely to still be active and energetic, so changes in behaviour, such as wandering or aggressive outbursts, can be more challenging.
- Younger people with dementia are often unwilling to give up driving, as this reduces independence. However, people with dementia should not drive and are unlikely to be able to get insurance following diagnosis.
- Behaviours can lead to issues such as arrests for shoplifting: this is less likely to be recognised as resulting from dementia than it would be with an older person.

Employment

It is likely that a younger person with dementia may be unable to continue working. Their partner may also have to leave work to become their carer, so a serious loss of income and changes in lifestyle can result.

They will not be in receipt of a state or occupational pension, so they need to ensure that they are claiming all the benefits that they are entitled to.

Legal and financial matters

Younger people with dementia are more likely to have financial commitments, such as mortgages. They are also more likely to have a living partner, so issues such as joint bank accounts need to be dealt with.

Plans need to be made to consider lasting power of attorney in relation to health and welfare or property and financial affairs. These arrangements are similar, but slightly different, for people living in Scotland.

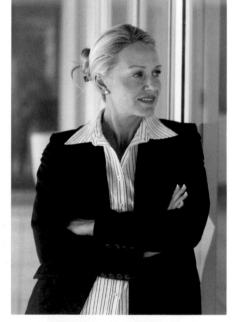

How do you think it would feel to have to give up work due to dementia at this age?

Activity

Research the facilities for younger people with dementia in your local area:

- Find out what is offered by local GPs, hospitals and Social Services.
- Check whether there are any local voluntary organisations or support groups for younger people with dementia or their carers.
- Find out how people can access the services and how many people use them.

The best place to start is with your own organisation, and work from there. Remember, the term 'younger people' in this context means anyone under the age of 65.

AC 207:3.2 and 209:3.1

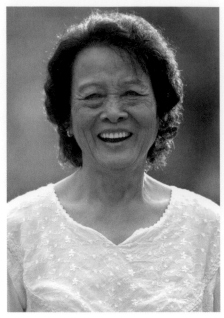

Did you know that vascular dementia is thought to be more common among Asian and Black Caribbean groups?

3.2 Needs and preferences of individuals from different ethnic origins

Everyone's experience of dementia is different and unique to them. However, there are similarities within some factors that influence the experience of different people: a person's ethnic and cultural background is one of these factors. It is important that you understand how dementia is viewed within the black and minority ethnic (BME) community and the likely impact of that on the way the condition is managed and supported.

The latest estimates in the government's dementia strategy, *Living Well with Dementia*, are that there are about 15,000 people from BME communities currently living with dementia. This is expected to rise considerably as people who arrived in the UK during the 1950s, 1960s and 1970s reach older age. There is little hard evidence about the frequency of dementia in various BME populations, but it is thought that vascular dementia is more common among Asian and Black Caribbean groups. This is because they are more likely to have the diseases that cause higher risks of dementia such as cardiovascular disease, diabetes and high blood pressure.

How dementia is viewed

Awareness of dementia seems to be low among Black Caribbean communities and, interestingly, there is no word for dementia in South Asian languages. There is a tendency to consider that the symptoms of dementia are part of normal ageing and to assume that nothing can be done. This can often mean that people only ask for help when dementia is quite advanced, giving a reduced opportunity for people to make choices and decisions about their support.

There is a stigma attached to dementia in all cultures, but this can be more obvious in some BME communities. For example, in some Asian religious groups dementia may be viewed as a punishment for past lives. In Black Caribbean communities, it is more likely to be viewed as a mental illness rather than as changes to the brain. In communities where there are arranged marriages, a family member with dementia is seen as affecting the marriage prospects of younger members. There is evidence that in Eastern European communities, the stigma of dementia is linked to previous experiences of persecution.

A study by Lawrence et al. in 2010, titled 'Threat to valued elements of life: the experience of dementia across three ethnic groups', compared the elements of life that were important to people with dementia. The study found that:

- white British people with dementia were most concerned about retaining independence for as long as possible
- Black Caribbean people were concerned about being a burden to their families
- Asian people valued family support, and were proud of it.

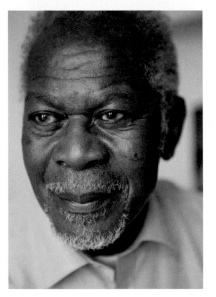

Are you surprised at the results of the study mentioned here?

Life histories

Life histories are very important when working with people from BME communities. They will help you make sure that you are responding to the person as an *individual* and not using racial or ethnic stereotypes to assess their needs.

Many of the people from BME communities who are developing dementia now were not born in the UK. This means that important parts of their lives will have taken place in another country, and the process of migration is likely to be a key memory.

In the future, there will be far more people from BME communities who were born in the UK, so their life histories will not have this element.

Carers

Research ('Dementia care-giving in black and Asian populations: reviewing and refining the research agenda' and 'Asian experiences of care-giving for older relatives with dementia: an exploration of barriers to uptake of support services') carried out among carers in BME communities shows that there is a very high expectation that women and adult children will undertake caring. Findings show that people in BME communities do not see themselves as 'carers' as such. The concept of caring for a family member is part of the obligations and duty of kinship. This is why people may be reluctant to seek support: they are concerned that external services will not meet the same standards as family care, or that they will be criticised within the community for using services rather than providing family support.

Increasingly, now, women from BME communities are working, so it is becoming more difficult for them to undertake traditional caring roles.

Working with people from different communities

The basic requirements of working well with people from backgrounds and cultures different to your own are the same regardless of the user group. Make sure that you find out information about the cultural and religious beliefs of the individual, and familiarise yourself with basic words in the person's language. Do not forget that people who speak English as a second language may lose the ability to speak it as their dementia progresses. Ensure that communication is undertaken in the language that a person can use and understand.

It is important that social activities are appropriate and that all cultural dietary needs are considered. Consultation with the person, their family and local community are important to be sure that you are providing a service that will meet the person's needs.

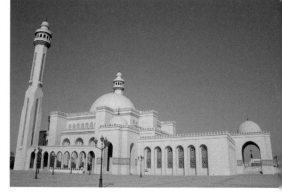

How much do you know about the cultural and religious beliefs of the people that you work with?

Activity

Research the services that are available in your area for people from BME communities (this will vary depending on where you live).

- Start with your own organisation. Then try voluntary groups, Social Services and health services.
- Include residential, day care services, domiciliary care services, specialist housing, advocacy, rights advice and befriending services.

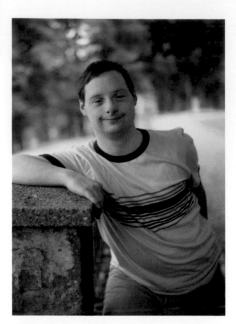

Were you aware of these statistics (right)?

3.3 Individuals with a learning disability

People with learning disabilities are living longer, and they are in better health than previously: this is because of advances in medical and social care. As a result, more people with a learning disability are living into older age and developing the conditions associated with ageing, including dementia.

Incidence of dementia in people with Down's syndrome

There is a known connection between Down's syndrome and dementia. People with Down's syndrome have a much higher chance of developing dementia at a younger age than the rest of the population, or than other people with different types of learning disability. The risk is three or four times higher than the general population. The most common form of dementia for people with Down's syndrome is Alzheimer's disease.

According to the Alzheimer's Society, the numbers of people with Down's syndrome who have Alzheimer's disease are estimated at:

- 1 in 50 of those aged 30–39
- 1 in 10 of those aged 40–49
- 1 in 3 of those aged 50–59
- more than half of those who live to 60 or over.

The reasons for this are not completely understood as yet, but it seems likely that the proteins that change the brain in Alzheimer's disease have a genetic link to the chromosome that causes Down's syndrome.

Incidence of dementia in people with other learning disabilities

The numbers of people with learning disabilities other than Down's syndrome who have dementia are estimated by the Alzheimer's Society to be:

- 1 in 10 of those aged 50–65
- 1 in 7 of those aged 65–75
- 1 in 4 of those aged 75–85
- nearly three-quarters of those aged 85 or over.

These figures show that there is a much higher incidence of younger people with a learning disability who develop dementia in comparison to the general population.

The different issues for people with learning disabilities

Many people with a learning disability will experience some of the same issues as younger people without a learning disability, but there are some differences:

- **There are some different signs and symptoms in the early stages**. For example, changes in behaviour are more likely to be noticed initially, rather than memory loss: people are reported as becoming withdrawn, or very stubborn and irritable. Epilepsy is more common among people with Down's syndrome than in the general population, but if a person only begins to have fits in later life, it is often a symptom of dementia.
- **People are less likely to receive an early diagnosis of dementia**. Health professionals or carers may not recognise the start of dementia, although there

is widespread awareness of the link between Alzheimer's disease and Down's syndrome.

- **People with Down's syndrome may have difficulty understanding the implications of a diagnosis of dementia, and find the changes in their own behaviour and abilities confusing and frustrating**. The person and/or their family are likely to require specific support to understand the changes, and to make sure they can access appropriate services after diagnosis and as dementia progresses.
- **There tends to be a more rapid progression of dementia**. The stages of dementia are the same for people with Down's syndrome, but the move into each stage may be quicker than for the general population.
- **People may already be in a supported living environment, or be supported by family**. As dementia develops, the changes may make it a challenge for the person to remain in their usual living environment, as additional support may be needed.
- **People may already have a communication plan**, depending on the severity and nature of the learning disability.
- **People may already have support in place** and regular contact with social work, community, day, residential or housing services.

Diagnosing dementia

Diagnosis will vary depending on the severity of the learning disability. Diagnosis of dementia is based on changes in behaviour rather than increasing memory loss and confusion, so it is important to take very detailed information from families or support workers to identify how and when changes began to happen.

There also needs to be a full health assessment to rule out any physical causes. People with a learning disability have an annual health check with their GP, so this is a good opportunity to examine any changes in behaviour that may indicate the start of dementia.

Working in a person-centred way

The principles of person-centred working apply in the same way to working with people with a learning disability. In fact, person-centred working was pioneered in the learning disability sector, so people should be used to making support plans and being in control of their own lives and support.

Many people with a learning disability will already have a life history and a personal profile. A diagnosis of dementia will mean that support plans should be reviewed so that the implications of the dementia diagnosis can be included. All of the important areas of person-centred work with people with dementia, such as history, local community, physical abilities, etc. are just as important when working with people with learning disabilities, and need to be looked at as part of a revised plan.

In the early stages, people will still be able to continue with most of the activities they have enjoyed: sport, walking, art, gardening, etc. should be encouraged. During the later stages, the range of current activities may be reduced and new ones introduced. Careful future planning can help to make smooth transitions as people progress through the stages of dementia, especially as this can be a quicker progression than for people without a learning disability.

Activity

Research the provision for people with a learning disability and dementia in your area.

Check to see if there are any specialist domiciliary, day services or residential services, and if any voluntary organisations offer any specialist services.

Even if you do not work in the field of learning disability, it is useful to know about specialist services.

Getting ready for assessment

DEM 207 is a knowledge-based unit. Each of the learning outcomes requires you to show your assessor that you have understood the learning. Your assessor may want you to do this through a written assignment or project, or you may be asked to prepare a presentation or a computer-based exercise. Sometimes, assessors will check your understanding through a professional discussion where you will answer questions that demonstrate that you understand all the learning.

This unit is all about equality, diversity and inclusion, so you will have to show that you understand why equality, diversity and inclusion matter, and how they affect the way services for people with dementia are delivered. Your assessor will want to see that you have understood how inclusive working makes dementia services more accessible. They will also want to see that you have understood how to recognise the diversity of people's individual and unique needs.

Person-centred working is also a key part of this unit. You may be able to use some of the assessment evidence from DEM 202 to meet the learning outcomes.

Some of the assessment criteria ask for specific things. When you are asked to explain, do not simply list or describe. Use words such as 'because', 'as a result of', 'so that' and 'in order to'. If you are explaining something, you must show that you understand the reasons for it.

DEM 209 is a competence-based unit that assesses knowledge and demonstration of skills. You will need to demonstrate in a workplace setting that you are able to work in a person-centred way with people and their carers and families. This means that you must show that you have found out as much as possible about the person you are supporting and know how their history influences their present. Your assessor will want to see that you have used life history to help you to meet a person's needs.

You will also need to show that you can support people from a range of ethnic and cultural backgrounds, and that you understand how dementia can be different for people who are younger or who have a learning disability.

You may be able to use some of the assessment evidence, particularly around person-centred working, from DEM 202.

Further reading and research

- Lawrence, V., Samsi, K., Banerjee, S., Morgan, C. and Murray, J. (2010) 'Threat to valued elements of life: the experience of dementia across three ethnic groups', *Gerontologist*.

- Milne A. and Chryssanthopoulou, C. (2005) 'Dementia care-giving in black and Asian populations: reviewing and refining the research agenda, *Journal of Community & Applied Social Psychology*, vol. 15, no. 5.

- Townsend, J. and Godfrey, M. (2001) 'Asian experiences of care-giving for older relatives with dementia: an exploration of barriers to uptake of support services', Leeds: Nuffield Institute for Health.

Chapter 5:
Approaches to enable rights and choices for individuals with dementia whilst minimising risks

Working with people with dementia means that you have to be able to balance rights and choices against risks to the personal safety of the person and others. The progressive nature of dementia can mean that people will have reduced capacity at some point. However, this does not mean that people lose capacity to make choices as soon as they are diagnosed with dementia, nor does it mean that they lose the capacity to make all decisions. People have rights regardless of the stage of their dementia, but they also have a right to be protected from serious harm, and sometimes this may mean that their freedoms have to be limited in order to ensure that they are not placing themselves at serious risk.

These are difficult balances to achieve. You will need to understand the issues that are behind some of these dilemmas if you are to be sure that you are taking the best possible actions to support people with dementia.

When you have achieved this unit you will:

■ understand key legislation and agreed ways of working that ensure the fulfilment of rights and choices of people with dementia while minimising risk of harm
■ understand how to maintain the right to privacy, dignity and respect when supporting people with dementia
■ support people with dementia to achieve their potential
■ be able to work with carers who are caring for people with dementia.

1: Legislation and ways of working that balance rights and choices and minimise risks

1.1 Key legislation

Basic human rights

In 1949, the United Nations Universal Declaration of Human Rights identified a set of basic rights that everyone should have. The Declaration sets out to promote and encourage acceptance of personal, civil, political, economic, social and cultural rights, which are only limited by the need to respect the rights and freedoms of others and the needs of morality, public order and general welfare. There are 30 articles in the Declaration and they cover all aspects of rights: the United Nations website, www.un.org, includes further detail.

These are rights that many people throughout the world can only hope for, and do not currently have. The United Nations has a Commission on Human Rights that works to promote the worldwide acceptance of these basic rights and to identify abuses and violations of human rights throughout the world. These basic human rights apply to everyone regardless of their position in life, their circumstances, or the way in which they are affected by any medical condition, including dementia.

Human Rights Act 1998

The United Kingdom (UK) protects human rights through an Act of Parliament. Most of the provisions of the Human Rights Act 1998 came into force on 2 October 2000. The Human Rights Act means that residents of the UK – this Act applies in England, Scotland, Wales and Northern Ireland – are entitled to seek help from the courts in the UK if they believe that their human rights have been infringed.

There is also a European Court of Human Rights that sits in Strasbourg and can be accessed as the highest court if people feel that they have not had justice from the UK courts.

The Human Rights Act applies to public bodies and to organisations that work on behalf of public bodies. Working in social care means that you are likely to work within the provisions of the Human Rights Act.

Table 5.1: Organisations subject to the Human Rights Act 1998

Organisation	Details
Residential homes or nursing homes	These perform functions which would otherwise be performed by a local authority. (People who fund their own care in residential homes are not covered by the Act.)
Charities	
Voluntary organisations	
Public services	This could include the privatised utilities, such as gas, electric and water companies, which will be affected by the provisions of this Act.

There are 16 rights (or Articles) protected under the Act:

1 The right to life.
2 The right to freedom from torture and inhuman or degrading treatment or punishment.
3 The right to freedom from slavery, servitude and forced or compulsory labour.
4 The right to liberty and security of person.
5 The right to a fair and a public trial within a reasonable time.
6 The right to freedom from retrospective criminal law and no punishment without law.
7 The right to respect for private and family life, home and correspondence.
8 The right to freedom of thought, conscience and religion.
9 The right to freedom of expression.
10 The right to freedom of assembly and association.
11 The right to marry and found a family.
12 The prohibition of discrimination in the enjoyment of convention rights.
13 The right to peaceful enjoyment of possessions and protection of property.
14 The right of access to an education.
15 The right of free elections.
16 The right not to be subjected to the death penalty.

These are broad rights and they can be interpreted for individuals. Within social care, making sure that people's rights are protected is a key part of your professional role. The code of practice for the regulating body for each of the UK countries is discussed in Section 1.2 on page 111, where you can also find information about how to ensure that your day-to-day work protects people's rights.

It is sometimes easy to forget that people with dementia also have the same human rights as everyone else. Just because someone is not always able to defend their rights or to make sure that the law is protecting them, does not mean that their rights are any less important or that they can be ignored.

Equality Act 2010

The Equality Act 2010 protects the rights of individuals and equality of opportunity.

It replaces many previous Acts, including:

• most of the provisions of the Disability Discrimination Acts 1995 and 2005
• the Equal Pay Act 1970
• the Sex Discrimination Act 1975
• the Race Relations Act 1976
• the Special Educational Needs and Disability Act 2001
• the Racial and Religious Hatred Act 2006
• the Equality Act 2006.

The Equality Act 2010 now protects different groups of people with just one Act. There are nine 'protected grounds' where the Act requires there to be equality:

1 Age
2 Disability

3 Gender

4 Race

5 Religion and belief

6 Pregnancy and maternity

7 Marriage and civil partnership

8 Sexual orientation

9 Gender reassignment.

Broadly, here is what the Act covers:

- The basic framework of protection against direct and indirect discrimination, harassment and victimisation in services and public functions, premises, work, education, associations and transport.

- Changing the definition of gender reassignment (sex change), by removing the requirement for medical supervision.

- Levelling up protection for people discriminated against because they have an association with someone who is protected under the Act, therefore providing new protection for people like carers.

- Clearer protection for breastfeeding mothers.

- Applying the European definition of indirect discrimination to all people protected under the Act.

- Extending protection from indirect discrimination to disability.

- Introducing a new concept of 'discrimination arising from disability'.

- Applying the same model as used in employment law to victimisation protection, so that people can be awarded damages if they have suffered as a result of the discrimination.

- Harmonising the thresholds for the duty to make reasonable adjustments for disabled people, so that all employers and providers of services have the same obligations.

- Extending protection from third-party harassment to all those protected by the Act.

- Making it more difficult for disabled people to be unfairly screened out when applying for jobs, by restricting the circumstances in which employers can ask job applicants questions about disability or health.

- Allowing 'what if?' examples to be used for direct gender pay discrimination.

- Making pay secrecy clauses unenforceable.

- Extending protection in private clubs to sex, religion or belief, pregnancy and maternity, and gender reassignment.

- Introducing new powers for employment tribunals to make recommendations that benefit the wider workforce.

- Making it possible for employers and providers of services to take positive action to support equality.

Although not all of the Act is relevant for everyone with dementia, it is relevant for younger people in the early stages of dementia, who may wish to continue working for as long as possible in order to retain their independence. This Act will ensure that employers must make reasonable adjustments to enable them to do their job, and cannot discriminate against them because of their condition.

The Act also protects people in their social and leisure activities. It means that where there is public access, places must make it possible for people with dementia to use the facilities.

Under the Act, a person has a disability if:

- they have a physical or mental impairment
- the impairment has a substantial and long-term adverse effect on their ability to perform normal day-to-day activities.

For the purposes of the Act, these three words/phrases have the following meanings:

- **Substantial** means more than minor or trivial.
- **Long term** means that the effect of the impairment has lasted, or is likely to last, for at least 12 months.
- **Normal day-to-day activities** include everyday things like eating, washing, walking and going shopping.

These definitions are important because it is very clear that most people with dementia are covered by the provisions of the Act and are protected from discrimination.

The Equality and Human Rights Commission has a statutory remit to promote and monitor human rights in the UK. The Commission protects and enforces equality across the nine 'protected grounds' under the Act.

Activity

Find out about the work of the Equality and Human Rights Commission in the UK, and how it applies to people with dementia.

Research any issues taken up by the Commission that have implications for people with dementia. For example, a recent investigation into home care found that older people were having their human rights breached. See what else you can find out.

Mental Capacity Act 2005

The Mental Capacity Act (MCA) sets out a framework for supporting people to make decisions, and lays out the ways in which people can be supported. The Act applies to England and Wales. Scotland has similar provision in the Adults with Incapacity (Scotland) Act (AIA).

The MCA is underpinned by five key principles:

1 **A presumption of capacity** – every adult has the right to make their own decisions and must be assumed to have capacity to do so unless it is proved otherwise.

2 **The right for individuals to be supported to make their own decisions** – people must be given all appropriate help, including advocates and support workers, before anyone concludes that they cannot make their own decisions.

3 **Individuals must retain the right to make what might be seen as eccentric or unwise decisions** –just because someone decides to do something that may seem foolish or risky, it does not mean that they are incapable of making decisions. After all, everyone does silly things sometimes.

4 Best interests – anything done for, or on behalf of, people without capacity must be in their best interests.

5 Least restrictive intervention – anything done for, or on behalf of, people without capacity should be the least restrictive of their basic rights and freedoms.

The Act sets out clearly how to establish if someone is incapable of taking a decision. The test to assess capacity is only in relation to a particular decision. No one can be deemed 'incapable' in general simply because of a medical condition or diagnosis.

The Act introduces a new criminal offence of ill treatment or neglect of a person who lacks capacity. A person found guilty of such an offence may be liable to imprisonment for a term of up to five years.

This Act is very important for people with dementia. Traditionally, there has been an assumption that people who have dementia have no capacity to make decisions. There was no legislation to protect them from having decisions made about their lives without their involvement or agreement. Since the implementation of the MCA and AIA (Scotland), people have to be given the opportunity to consider and make decisions for themselves, wherever possible. The Act is very specific that even if a decision appears unwise or eccentric, people still have a right to make it. For example, a person may decide to spend a large sum of money on a bicycle, even though they have poor mobility and cannot ride it. As long as they have capacity, they can buy a bike if they want to.

The principle that incapacity should be related to a specific instance is also very important. It can never be assumed that, because someone has dementia, they cannot make any decisions. Someone may be incapable of deciding when to take their medication because they have no idea of time. That does not mean that they cannot make a decision about whether to sell their home: they may be very clear that selling their home is something they do not want to do. It is the decision-making process – and the person's ability to go through the process – that is looked at under the Act, not the outcome of the decisions a person takes.

The assessment of capacity is the responsibility of the person who requires a decision. For example, if the question is about medical consent, then the health professional concerned needs to make the assessment. If it is about moving into residential care, then it is the social worker's responsibility. In the case of major decisions, or where there is doubt, the professional concerned will usually refer to a psychiatrist or psychologist for a second opinion. Major decisions are matters such as selling a home, agreeing to a course of medical treatment or moving into residential care. Day-to-day matters are issues such as choosing what to wear, or what to eat or whether to go out for a walk.

The test to assess capacity looks at the functions of decision making. The Act states that to decide whether an individual has the capacity to make a particular decision, you must first assess whether they have 'an impairment of, or a disturbance in the functioning of, the mind or brain', and, if so, whether the impairment or disturbance is sufficient that the person lacks the capacity to make a particular decision.

The person will be unable to make the particular decision if, after appropriate help and support to make the decision, they cannot:

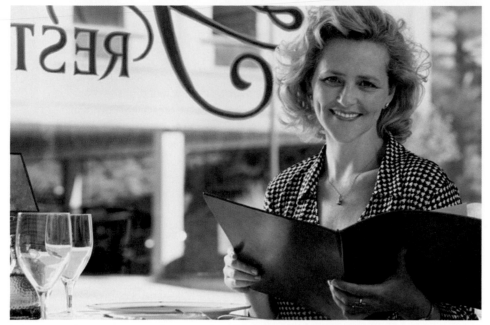

It is up to the person to choose what they would like to eat.

1 understand the information relevant to the decision
2 retain the information relevant to the decision
3 use, or weigh, the information
4 communicate the decision (by any means).

Adults with Incapacity (Scotland) Act

The AIA (Scotland) shares the same principles as the MCA and has the same criteria for judging capacity. Anyone authorised to make decisions on behalf of someone with impaired capacity must apply the following principles:

- **Benefit** – any action or decision taken must benefit the person and only be taken when that benefit cannot reasonably be achieved without it.

- **Least restrictive option** – any action or decision taken should be the minimum necessary to achieve the purpose. It should be the option that restricts the person's freedom as little as possible.

- **Take account of the wishes of the person** – when deciding if an action or decision is to be made, account must be taken of the present and past wishes and feelings of the person. Some people may not be capable of taking a particular decision, but will be able to express their wishes and feelings clearly.

- **The person must be offered help to communicate their views.** This might mean using memory aids, pictures, non-verbal communication, a speech and language therapist, or support from an independent advocate.

- **Consultation with relevant others** – the Act lists those who should be consulted whenever practicable and reasonable. It includes the person's primary carer, nearest relative, named person, attorney or guardian (if there is one).

- **Encourage the person to use existing skills and develop new skills**.
  In Scotland, if someone lacks the capacity to make a decision, then a welfare guardian will be appointed – this can be a relative, friend or social worker.

Think about a decision you have taken.

Look at each of the four parts of the capacity test. Make notes about how you took your decision and link your decision-making process to each part of the capacity assessment. Can you see how you followed the process of reaching a decision?

For example, you might have been making a decision about a new job, buying a computer or moving house. Any of those decisions would involve you going through a process before finally deciding.

Think about how decisions are made, and how the decision-making process applies to the people you support.

Deprivation of Liberty Safeguards

Safeguards for the MCA were introduced in 2009 following a court case about a young man who was detained in hospital without giving, or refusing, his consent. He lacked the capacity to willingly consent or refuse to be in hospital.

In the light of this case, the Safeguards were introduced so that assessments must be carried out before anyone can be detained in a hospital, a residential care home, or any facility.

The concept of deprivation of liberty can cover many different situations. Courts have been involved in several different cases, including:

- a patient being restrained in order to admit them to hospital
- medication being given against a person's will
- staff having complete control over a patient's care or movements for a long period
- staff taking all decisions about a patient, including choices about assessments, treatment and visitors
- staff deciding whether a patient can be released into the care of others, or to live elsewhere
- staff refusing to discharge a person into the care of others
- staff restricting a person's access to their friends or family.

If a facility wishes to use any form of restraint, very strict procedures must be followed.

A residential care facility must contact Social Services, who will arrange for a specially trained best interests assessor to decide if the deprivation of liberty is justified. There are clear guidelines for the assessor to follow, and a set of criteria that the person must meet. If the assessor is satisfied, then they will agree to an authorisation for the person. There must also be agreement from a mental health assessor, who must be a doctor (usually a psychiatrist or geriatrician). An authorisation is made for the shortest possible time, but can be up to a year.

People who have their liberty restricted must have a relevant person's representative (RPR). Usually this will be a family member or friend, but where this is not possible, they will have the services of an independent mental capacity advocate (IMCA). The role of the RPR is to ensure that the person's rights are respected and that they understand, as far as possible, about how their liberty is being restricted. All of those involved with the person are required to ensure that the RPR has all the information about the decision and ongoing support of the person.

> **Activity**
>
> Find out about Deprivation of Liberty Safeguards (DoLS) in your workplace.
>
> Have any authorisations been applied for? If so, what were the circumstances? If not, ask colleagues about any Safeguards they have been involved with.

Mental Health Act 2007

The Mental Health Act 2007 came into force in 2008 and made some changes to the Mental Health Act 1983.

The Act uses the term **mental disorder**. Within the Act, dementia is considered to be a mental disorder, and therefore the Act can apply to people with dementia.

People with dementia can be detained in a hospital under the Mental Health Act if they are considered to be behaving in a way that causes a danger to themselves or others. The 2007 Act allows people to have a guardian appointed to take decisions on their behalf, and to ensure that they comply with any requirements in relation to their health. A guardian can decide where someone has to live and make sure that they attend appointments.

The **nearest relative** looks after the interests of the person. One of the new provisions in the Act is that a nearest relative can include a civil partner.

Usually, a list is followed, and the nearest person in the list is considered to be the nearest relative.

This may be the person's:

- husband, wife or civil partner
- son or daughter
- father or mother
- brother or sister
- grandparent
- grandchild
- uncle or aunt
- nephew or niece.

It may also be someone (not a relative) whom the person has lived with for at least the last five years.

Another new provision in the Act is that anyone who is detained under the Mental Health Act can challenge the person who is considered to be their nearest relative. For example, someone may have a son who they have not seen for a long time, but he is legally the nearest relative. They may also have a niece who visits them daily. Previously, it would not have been possible for the niece to be designated as the nearest relative, but now the person can request it.

> **Key terms**
>
> **Mental disorder** – this term is used in the Mental Health Act 2007. Within the Act, dementia is considered to be a mental disorder.
>
> **Nearest relative** – the person who looks after the interests of the person.

The nearest relative can request that someone is detained in hospital, object to a guardian, discharge the person from hospital, and apply to a tribunal for someone to be discharged.

A court can change the designated nearest relative under certain circumstances if they have a request from a healthcare professional or the person themselves.

This could be done if it is considered that the nearest relative is:

- trying to discharge someone without sufficient regard for their welfare or the welfare of others
- unreasonably objecting to a guardianship order or detention for treatment
- unable to fulfil their role due to illness.

Professionals

Anyone who is detained in hospital under the Mental Health Act can have access to an **independent mental health advocate (IMHA)**, who can explain their rights. An IMHA is someone who can explain a person's rights and how to challenge a section decision. Advocates have access to the person's medical records and operate independently from the hospital.

People who have been found to lack capacity under the Mental Capacity Act can be assigned an **independent mental capacity health advocate (IMCA)**. Their role is to act in the person's best interests if they have been at risk of harm and are subject to safeguarding procedures.

An **approved mental health practitioner** is involved in decisions about whether someone should be detained under the Act. They are also involved in decisions about appointing a guardian. They are usually a social worker, but can be another mental health professional (such as a community psychiatric nurse) who is trained and approved to perform this role.

A **responsible clinician** is the health professional in charge of the person's care in the hospital. This is normally a doctor but they can be another health professional, such as a psychologist, social worker, mental health nurse or occupational therapist, who has been approved to perform this role.

Managing risks in the workforce

The workforce that supports vulnerable groups, like people with dementia, always presents some risks. Some people may try to take advantage of people with dementia for personal gain. Others may want to be in a position of power and can exploit or harm those people whom they should be supporting.

There are organisations responsible for checking the suitability of people to work in social care.

In England, Wales and Northern Ireland this is done by the Independent Safeguarding Authority (ISA), which maintains the list of people barred from working with children and young people, and also the list of those barred from working with vulnerable adults.

In Scotland, the Protecting Vulnerable Groups (PVG) scheme has the same lists being maintained by Disclosure Scotland. The same organisation is also responsible for identifying the criminal records of people who want to work with any vulnerable groups. In Northern Ireland, these checks are carried out by Access NI, and in England and Wales by the Criminal Records Bureau (CRB).

Changes in how these risks are managed will take place in 2012 under the Protection of Freedoms Bill, due to become law in May 2012.

The Bill will:

- combine the ISA and CRB
- provide a system of 'portable' criminal records checks
- reduce the number of people who have to be subject to checks.

1.2 Ways of working

Wherever you work, there will be policies and procedures about how to make sure that people's rights are protected and that you are working within the relevant legislation.

If you are working as a personal assistant directly employed by someone with dementia, you are an example of how that person is exercising their rights and choice. By choosing to employ someone directly, they are maintaining control over how and when their support is delivered. However, it is still your responsibility to carry out your duty of care: to make sure that your actions are promoting your employer's rights and that you are working within the law and national guidelines.

If you are employed by an organisation, there will be policies and processes in place to make sure that people are able to exercise their rights to make choices about how they live and what they do.

Your professional responsibility is to act within the **code of practice** of the regulator for your country. This lays out the duties and expectations for everyone who works in the sector.

Having codes of practice is important. By working with people who have dementia, you work with some of the most vulnerable people in society, who have a right to expect a certain standard of work and a certain standard of moral and ethical behaviour.

In order to work in social work anywhere in the UK, and in social care in some parts (soon to be all) of the UK, there is a requirement to be registered. This means having, or working towards, a certain minimum level of qualification, and agreeing to work within the code of practice that sets out the behaviour that is required. Employers have to ensure that everyone who works for them is registered and eligible to work in social work or social care.

At the moment, only social care practitioners in Scotland and Wales are registered, but England and Northern Ireland will be following in the near future. In any event, abiding by the relevant code of practice is a good way of making sure that your practice is following ethical and professional guidelines.

1.3 Making decisions

The process of decision making and the legal position under the Mental Capacity Act 2005 has been discussed earlier in this chapter. The principles of the Act include the idea that everyone is assumed to have the capacity to make decisions unless there is evidence that they do not.

It is also important to remember that the Act states that people can only be found to lack capacity for a specific decision. This does not mean that they are incapable of making any decisions. For example, someone may be very capable of deciding what to eat or what to wear, but may not be able to manage their finances.

People with dementia may need support to make decisions, but that does not mean that they should not make them. All possible support should be provided: this could include support with communication, such as flash cards, or it may mean using an advocate to explain the person's wishes. Making decisions is part of every person's life: it gives people dignity and is part of our rights as a human being. Being in control of our own lives is good for our self-esteem and overall well-being; so being able to make decisions for as long as possible is very important.

The following comments are from people with dementia about how they feel when decisions are made for them:

> *It sometimes seemed that the minute my back was turned, something else would be done without any consultation and always with the comment that it was for my own good and that I had been told what was going on.*
>
> *When my family said 'you can't go' it made me angry. I am capable of doing so much. I have forethought and foresight to know if I can't do a challenge.*

Advance decisions

Some people may want to prepare certain decisions in advance, before the dementia progresses to the point where they are no longer able to do so. Advance decisions can be made and recorded: they may concern certain types of medical treatment, or where a person wishes to be supported to live. They may also identify priorities for how they want future care and support to be provided, and also how they wish their end-of-life care to be given.

Case study

Marjorie is in the early stages of dementia. She has researched what is likely to happen and understands how the stages of dementia are likely to progress.

She is currently very able to make all her own decisions, and she has done so. She has chosen to remain in her own home and is supported by a mix of family and friends. For the moment, she does not need the support of professional carers, but she has decided to go to the day centre for a day each week, as she wants to get to know other people in a similar situation to herself. She is also happy to spend time on her own and still enjoys meeting up with friends and listening to music, watching old films and gardening. She no longer knits clothes, as she finds the patterns confusing, but has been knitting some squares for the local church.

Marjorie has sat down with her children and prepared some advance decisions about what she wants to happen later. She has decided that she will only go into residential care at the point where she is a risk at home. She feels that her son and daughter will be able to decide that if she is unable to. Her preference would be to remain at home with professional support. At this

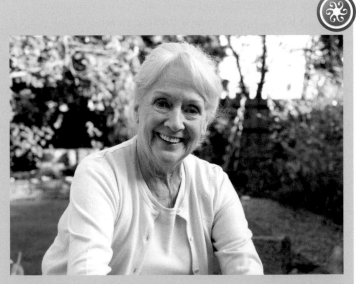

point, she does not think that she would want to be resuscitated if she were to develop a life-threatening condition.

1 Do you think it is helpful for Marjorie to write down her decisions in advance?

2 Who will benefit from her doing this?

3 How do you think Marjorie feels about being able to do this?

These are all helpful ways in which people can be involved in decisions and have their wishes taken into account, even after they have passed the stage of being able to make decisions independently.

1.4 Best interests of an individual with dementia

The MCA requires that any decisions that have to be taken on behalf of an individual because they lack capacity must be 'in the person's best interests'. The person's interests take priority over others' interests, such as family, other patients or residents, or the general public.

The MCA does not set out a process for making decisions, as the types of decisions are so varied. It does set out what needs to be taken into consideration in the 'best interests' checklist. Anyone who is taking a decision in the best interests of someone who lacks capacity must comply with this checklist:

- **The decision must not be made merely on the basis of the person's age or appearance**. In other words, a proper assessment of capacity must have been carried out.

- **The person's behaviour should not lead to assumptions about what might be in their best interests**. All aspects of a decision and potential consequences should be considered, and reasons for any behaviour must also be considered.

- **All relevant circumstances need to be considered**. All aspects of someone's life and present circumstances should be taken into account.

- **Is the person likely to regain capacity? Can the decision wait?** Obviously, this is unlikely in the case of someone with dementia, although the question must be asked.

- **Involve the person in the decision making as much as possible. Even though it has been determined that the individual lacks capacity to make this decision, their views need to be considered and the process needs to include them as far as possible**. All efforts to use various means of communication should be used to try to get the person's views as far as possible.

- **If the decision concerns life-sustaining treatment, the decision must not be based on a desire to bring about death. The MCA cannot be used for the purposes of euthanasia**. In other words, if a person is on life support, best interest decision making cannot be used to decide to end the life support.

- **The decision maker must consider the person's past and present wishes, beliefs and values that would influence their decision making if they had capacity, and any other factors the person would take into consideration if making their own decision**. This is where any advance decisions can be useful: they can help the decision maker to understand what the person is most likely to want.

- **The decision maker must take into account the views of anyone caring for the person or interested in their welfare: this includes paid and informal carers. The decision maker must consult, if possible, anyone who has a Lasting Power of Attorney or who is a deputy appointed by the Court of Protection**. All of those who are involved with the person should be included if at all possible. Sometimes people will have useful information that was not known previously, or they may have an insight that others have missed.

It is important to remember that people are being involved to get their views of what is likely to be in the best interests of the person: it is not about what is in the best interests of carers.

1.5 Least restrictive way to provide care and support

One of the principles of behaving in someone's best interests is that whatever action needs to be taken, it must give people as much freedom as possible, and must limit their lives as little as possible.

Here are two examples.

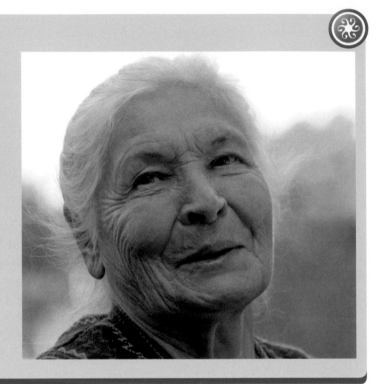

Case studies

Tom

Tom likes to go out walking every day, but he gets lost. The last time he was picked up by the police, he was walking down the approach road to the motorway. Tom is moving towards an advanced stage of dementia, but becomes very distressed if he does not get to walk each day.

A decision will need to be taken in Tom's best interests about if, or how, he is able to go for a daily walk.

June

June lives at home and has support from family and professional carers. She has always been adamant that she wished to remain in her own home, and she made this clear in her advanced decisions and care priorities when she was able.

Her dementia is progressing. She has left the gas turned on but unlit on several occasions recently. Neighbours are supportive but concerned, as her house is terraced.

In Tom's case, the least restrictive option would be for him to have his daily walk with an assistant, who could support him and ensure that he returns safely. Tom could be made to stay in, but that would be very restrictive and definitely a decision he would oppose if he were able.

In June's situation, the options being discussed are:

- a move to a residential home
- a move to extra care housing
- replacing the gas cooker with an electric one
- turning off the gas to the cooker and providing prepared meals for the microwave.

The social worker and June's family decided on the last option. This was felt to be the least restrictive way to support June.

2: How to maintain the right to privacy, dignity and respect

Everyone is entitled to be treated with dignity and respect: this means all aspects of life, from support with personal care to how people want to be addressed. It is also about listening to what people have to say and being interested in them. Sometimes people with dementia do not get the respect they deserve, nor do they get treated with dignity because it is all too easy to assume that 'they won't know'.

Not only is this far from the truth, but even if it were accurate for some people, being unaware of your surroundings does not make poor and unprofessional attitudes acceptable. In fact, people who struggle to grasp the world around them deserve even more care and consideration.

2.1 Privacy for personal care

Everyone has a right to have some space where they can be alone if they wish. Sometimes they may want to be private just to have some time to themselves. On other occasions it may be because they are having personal care or medical treatment. It is also important that people have privacy if they want to talk to a professional and have confidential information to discuss.

Ideally, people should be able to manage their personal care independently and in private. However, this is not always the case and some people with dementia may need a degree of assistance. How much someone can manage unaided is likely to change over time as the dementia progresses. This will need to be kept under constant review with the person and any family or friend carers.

Sometimes it can be risky for the person to manage personal care for themselves unsupervised. For example, someone may struggle to remain focused on what they are doing and forget to get fully dressed, or forget to check the temperature of a bath or shower. People may be unable to recall the right order for putting on clothes, or may forget to clean themselves properly after using the toilet. In the early stages of dementia, this is less likely to be a problem, but as time passes it is important to change levels of support.

If support is needed and agreed, then you must work in a sensitive way. Try to empathise with the person's situation. Simple actions can maximise privacy and

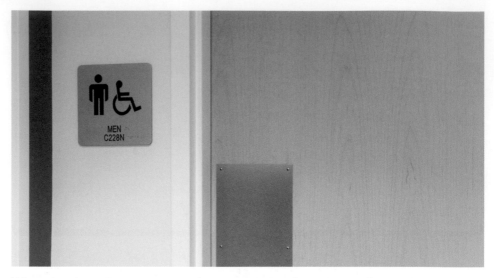

What simple actions can you take to maximise the privacy of a person with dementia?

make all the difference – for example, knocking on the door before entering the room. It can be more difficult in a hospital setting where there may only be a curtain to maintain privacy. In this situation, you can make sure that there are no gaps and alert the person by calling their name and asking permission to enter before opening the curtains.

If someone is being supported with personal care at home, they may be unable to use their bathroom (for example, if it is upstairs and they have limited mobility). In this scenario, you can ensure that privacy is maintained by closing curtains or blinds and making sure that the room door is closed.

Modesty is greatly valued by some religions and cultural groups. Talk to the person and their family in order to check the level of privacy required by someone's religion or culture when personal care is being undertaken.

If someone requires full support for personal care, maximum privacy can still be maintained. If the person needs help with an assisted wash or a blanket bath, ensure that they remain covered as much as possible by using extra towels or a warm sheet.

Reflect

Imagine that you are a patient in a hospital and you share a bay with five other people. There are people of the opposite sex on the ward in other bays. You have had an operation and are unable to manage your own personal care, so you need someone to help you.

How would you feel? How would you like to be supported?

2.2 Showing respect for physical space

Space is important to us all. The amount of personal space you need can change depending on the environment in which you live. For example, if you live in a house with other members of your family, you may consider that a bedroom is the minimum amount of space you need to call your own. If you live alone, you may feel that you need the whole house in order to feel that you have sufficient space. On the other hand, if you are staying on a hospital ward for a long time, your personal space can shrink to a locker by your bed.

Whatever it is and whatever size, having personal, physical space is an important part of well-being: somewhere you feel that you are in charge and in control, and others cannot enter without permission.

Respecting people's physical space recognises a person's right to be treated with dignity and to have their rights as an individual recognised and valued. Doing this includes simple actions such as:

- knocking before going into a person's room
- always giving someone their handbag to look for something rather than you rummaging through it
- making sure that people can keep their personal belongings where they are easily accessible.

Moving into a residential setting can be difficult. Many older people have spent time living alone, or with just one other person. Learning to live in a space surrounded by many other people can make the need for personal space very important.

Having a room where a person can go and know that they won't be disturbed can make the difference between someone settling and feeling positive about their living environment, and someone becoming very agitated and distressed.

Creating spaces, perhaps alcoves or private areas, or using furniture if alterations are not possible, can offer relief from stress and anxiety for people in a group living situation.

2.3 Showing respect for social or emotional space

The physical space between people usually indicates how close the relationship is. When talking to strangers, we may keep an arm's length apart. The ritual of shaking hands indicates that you have been introduced: you may come closer. When you are friendly with someone, you may accept the person coming even closer to you. Close family and sexual partners are able to be closest.

People in different cultures have different assumptions about how close people should be when they are talking. People in some cultures are much more inclined to touch each other than in others. For example, in Arab cultures, men will hug and kiss on meeting. This is not generally done in the UK, but it is slowly becoming more acceptable among younger people.

When people have dementia, the usual distances may be slightly different. Evidence shows that many people with dementia respond well to closeness and often to touch, especially if people are confused and disorientated. However, do not assume that everyone with dementia wants to be touched, or have their hand held or stroked. You should always check that someone is comfortable with being close and with being touched.

Respecting someone's personal space is very important when you are working. If you enter someone's personal space without asking or explaining, it is disrespectful and people may feel very uncomfortable with it.

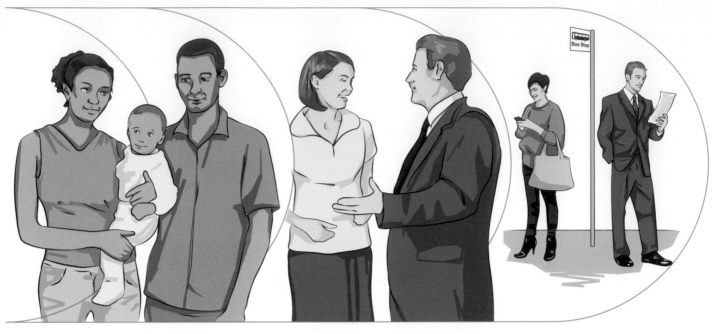

| Intimate zone (touching) | Personal zone (Less than 1 metre) | Social zone (1-2 metres) | Public zone (2 metres +) |

Figure 5.1: Does this work for you?

Research has shown that there are 'zones' of distance within which we are comfortable. These are:

- the **public zone** – strangers tend to maintain a distance, usually more than about two metres, unless squashed together on a train or in a crowd
- the **social zone** – acquaintances can come slightly closer
- the **personal zone** – friends are accepted into this zone
- the **intimate zone** – usually reserved for close family and partner.

Make sure that you check you are operating in a space that is acceptable to the person you are supporting. Do not just assume that contact or closeness will be acceptable.

2.4 Using an awareness of life history and culture to maintain dignity

Chapters 2 and 3 looked in depth at the importance of creating life histories for the people you support. The process of developing a history helps you to see the *person* rather than the dementia, and to recognise that dementia is about much more than a disease.

As we mentioned earlier in the book, Tom Kitwood was one of the first people to recognise that the progress of each individual's dementia is dependent on many factors, but one of them is the person's own background and life history.

2.5 The benefits of knowing about a person's life history

Everyone is entitled to be treated with dignity and respect. This is easier to do with someone that you know about, where you have understood and valued the contribution they have made throughout their life.

Finding out someone's background is fascinating and shows you the way they have contributed to society through their work, bringing up a family, or being active in their local community. Undertaking life story work, especially alongside family and friends, helps you to see the person beneath the dementia, and therefore makes it much easier to ensure that they are given the dignity and respect they deserve.

Case study

Dalston is in the late stages of dementia. He appears not to know people, but does sometimes smile when his daughter comes to visit. He struggles with communication, but can sometimes communicate using picture cards.

He often likes to look at the photographs in his life story book and will sometimes laugh and point to a particular picture. When working on his life story book, staff were amazed to hear from his family and friends how he had come to the UK from Jamaica in the 1950s with his young wife. They had settled in London, where he worked as a bus driver for many years.

In his spare time, he devoted himself to starting a local youth club that offered many sports and activities in the deprived area in which they lived. The family was never rich, but the children were always well fed and clothed, discipline was firm, and good behaviour was expected. Dalston devoted many years of his life to working voluntarily with young people. He motivated many young people away from a life of crime and encouraged them to get an education and find work. He was very well respected among the young people in the area and received an honour presented by the Queen for his work with young people.

All three of his children have degrees and they are all in professional jobs. Even though Dalston worked very hard to put them all through university, he always found time for his youth work.

All the staff found that they had a different view of Dalston once they knew about his life and his achievements. His daughter

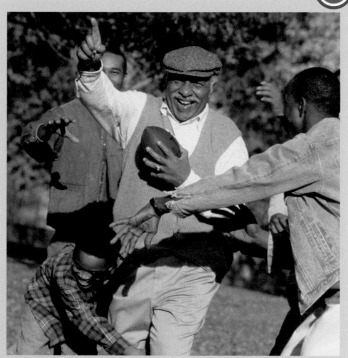

commented that she was so happy now that the staff knew about her dad as he really was, and not just like he was now.

1   How did working on the life story book help Dalston to be treated with dignity?

2   What might have happened if no one had known about his life?

Knowing about people's interests also helps to ensure that individual activities are organised that reflect people's interests and skills. In Dalston's case, staff were able to use pictures with a sporting theme to interest him: he was often seen drawing pictures copied from photographs of football games and boxing matches. He loved cricket and staff would sometimes take him to the local cricket ground where he would watch for a while, usually smiling, before losing concentration.

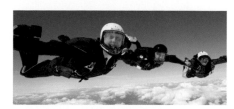

How much do you know about what the people you support have done in the past?

3: Support people with dementia to achieve their potential

3.1 Physical environment

Where people live has just as much impact on well-being as *how* people live.

When someone has dementia, living in the right environment, with well-thought-out design, can make a significant difference to how well they can function. Considerable work has been undertaken by architects and designers to look at how to get the best environment for people with dementia.

There are some basic, internationally agreed principles that design should:

- compensate for impairments
- maximise independence
- enhance self-esteem and confidence
- be understandable and not confusing
- reinforce people's identity
- not be over stimulating.

Compensate for impairments

The thinking behind the idea that design should compensate for impairments is that an impairment only becomes a disability if the design of a living space does not overcome the impairment.

For example, people with dementia may have impaired memory. Creating an open-plan design where all areas can be seen, and eating areas and sitting areas are easily located, can assist people to feel comfortable and familiar with their

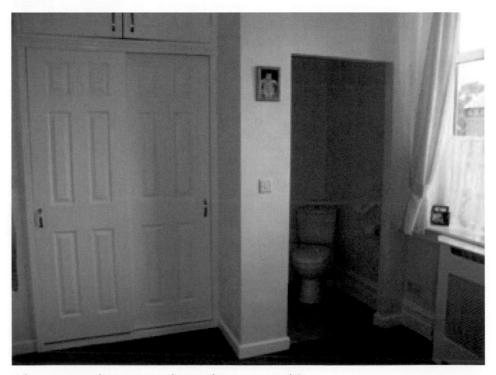

What en-suite layouts are there where you work?

surroundings. Another helpful design feature is always to have bathroom doors in the same colour, and a good contrast to the surrounding walls. Signs should be large and clear, and in en-suite bathrooms the toilet should be clearly visible from the bed. These may sound like small details, but they all assist people to live well with dementia.

People with dementia are also likely to have impaired reasoning and find it difficult to make judgements and to process information. People can lose the ability to tell the difference between colours, so sharp contrasts are important. Difficulties in recognising colours usually start with blues, purples and greens. Reds, oranges and yellows tend to be recognised for longest, so these can be good colours to choose.

Other helpful design features include:

- having contrasts between surfaces and objects
- having a clear contrast between floor and wall finishes, and between handrails, grabrails and the walls behind
- light switches contrasting clearly with the background
- toilet seats contrasting with the toilet, which in turn contrasts with the background floor and wall tiling.

A sharp contrast in flooring can be perceived as a step by people with dementia. So similar colours in flooring should be used, but different textures between hard floor and carpet can show different areas.

When people have impaired orientation, it has been found that architectural features, rather than colour, can often be the most helpful way for people to find their way around. Curved walls, or different textures for wall coverings or features, such as clocks or plants, should be individual so that people find it easier to know where they are.

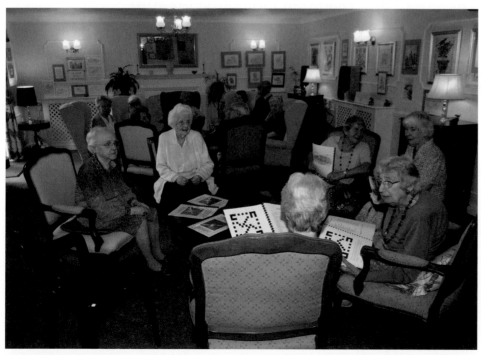

What other design features could improve the living environment for people with dementia?

Maximise independence

A well-designed environment can help people to make the most of their independence by giving them the opportunity to safely explore and move around the building.

Many people with dementia like to walk. Providing indoor or outdoor areas for safe walking can help people to be independent and make their own choices about when and where they will walk. Areas such as exit doors can be painted to match surrounding walls, and removing features such as door frames can reduce the risks of people wandering out of the premises.

Enhance self-esteem and confidence

People's self-esteem and confidence can be improved by supporting them to maintain their skills.

Adjustable-height kitchen work surfaces and careful thought being given to the kitchen layout can help with this. The option for residents to contribute to the running of their own household by undertaking everyday tasks is important in maintaining a continuation of their everyday life. In some residential facilities, the kitchenettes in the care home households are accessible to residents, and meals, snacks and drinks are made by the residents and staff together. Dementia should not prevent people from being active in their community. Residential or extra care facilities should be able to use garden areas and community rooms for clubs and groups to meet.

Be understandable and not confusing

Environment need to be clear and simple to understand. Lots of different colours and textures can be very confusing. Signs need to be clear and use pictures as well as written words.

Recognise and reinforce individual identity

Rooms that help to maintain people's identity are important. People should be able to have their own belongings around them. The opportunity to have memory boxes around the door area helps people to recognise their own room and also gives others information about who lives there.

Levels of stimulation

It is important that there is a calm and relaxed atmosphere in a living environment for people with dementia. Too many different 'busy' and noisy features can add to confusion and anxiety. It is easy for people with dementia to be over stimulated by too many bright colours, bright and harsh lighting, and too much noise. Thought needs to be given to 'quiet' floor coverings and to making sure that there is the opportunity to access quiet and peaceful areas.

Activity

Look again at the design principles in the bulleted list on page 120.

Now apply each one of them to your workplace. How well does your workplace fit these criteria? Is there more that could be done? What could be improved, and how would you go about it?

Make notes and draw some plans of what you would like to do. You could research and put together photographs of rooms and designs that you think would improve the living environment of the people you support.

If you work with people in their own homes, design a new residential or extra care facility.

3.2 Social environment

Supporting people with dementia means providing a social environment that:

- encourages them to do as much as they can for themselves
- ensures that they make their own choices about how they wish to live
- makes sure that they do not have routines imposed on them.

The overall atmosphere should be calm and relaxed, and provide people with a feeling of warmth, security and caring. This type of environment is likely to make people with dementia feel less anxious and confused, more orientated and focused, and therefore better able to participate and maintain skills and intellectual functioning.

3.3 Active involvement

Even though a caring and secure environment is important, that does not mean that people should have everything done for them. The ability to make choices and take risks is an important part of supporting people to reach their potential. Everyone should be encouraged to do as much as they possibly can for themselves. It is likely that the more that people with dementia are encouraged, the more they will be able to achieve.

Participating in activities with others and achieving goals usually helps people to feel good about themselves, and improves confidence and self-esteem. How we value ourselves is vital to our sense of well-being. Feeling good and feeling confident are important ways of improving people's general and emotional health. This is no less true for people with dementia. Feeling self-confident and independent is just as important.

It is tempting to do things *for* people because it may seem easier, quicker, less difficult and helpful to the person. In fact, doing tasks for people is far from helpful. It results in people becoming de-skilled and increases dependency. Increasing dependency also decreases people's confidence, self-esteem and sense of well-being, resulting in people becoming more depressed and isolated. It is a vicious circle.

Encourage people to undertake as much of their personal care as they can possibly manage, including:

- hygiene
- managing their own appearance
- choosing clothes
- keeping themselves clean.

Obviously, the level of ability to do this will vary with the stage of dementia and will change over time, but people should always do the absolute maximum that they can.

Working *with* people to support them where there are things that they really cannot do for themselves is so much better than taking over, doing tasks for people and making them dependent on you.

> **Reflect**
>
> Think about someone you support.
>
> Identify a task or activity that is carried out *for* them:
>
> - Why are they unable to do this task themselves?
> - Is there anything more that could be done to support them to do this for themselves?

3.4 Attitudes of others

The way that people with dementia are viewed and treated by various groups of people can make a major difference to their well-being and the achievement of their potential.

Professionals

Some professionals may still regard a person with dementia as having a disease, with symptoms that need to be managed, rather than as an *individual* with a different way of seeing the world, and as a *person* who is better at managing some aspects of their life than others. This attitude can lead to people not being able to do as much as they are capable of. Their abilities are not recognised, and people are not enabled to make choices and take risks because professionals are not willing to support risky courses of action.

Families

Families may want to protect people who they see as vulnerable and in need of care, and may have many concerns about the risks to loved ones of making choices and taking risks. Do not jump to the conclusion that families are being difficult or obstructive: usually people believe that they are doing their best for their relatives by protecting them and by reducing risks.

Working in partnership with people and their families to help them get used to person-centred approaches and to see the benefits of person-centred working may be a slow process, and one that needs to be taken gently. However, the long-term benefits of people with dementia being able to participate fully in their own lives are worth it.

Local communities

The support of local communities is important, particularly when people with dementia live in their own homes. Having a supportive neighbourhood group who will share in the support of a person with dementia can make all the difference between someone being able to stay in their own home and having to move into residential care. Examples of support include watching out for them, helping if they see them at the shops, and checking whether their front door is left open or the lights have been left on. There are always risks that someone with dementia will be exploited by people in the community, but there are also great opportunities to support people to live their lives as they want to. Careful monitoring of community support helps to reduce risks and makes it more likely that people will be able to do the things they want to, in their own way.

4: Working with carers of people with dementia

4.1 Anxieties common to carers

There are over six million carers in the UK. Not all of those are caring for someone with dementia, but many are.

Generally, people who care for relatives or friends do so willingly and with love. Some are doing it because they feel they have been forced into the situation, but this is rare. Caring is hard work and can be very stressful. Looking after someone with dementia is very demanding and can be frustrating and infuriating, especially as family carers do not get to go home at the end of a shift.

4.2 Legal rights for carers

Scotland has a Charter of Rights for people with dementia and their carers. Here are their broad rights:

- People with dementia and their carers have the right to participate in decisions which affect their human rights.
- Those responsible for the care and treatment of people with dementia should be held accountable for the respect, protection and fulfilment of their human rights.
- Non-discrimination and equality.
- Empowerment to know their rights and how to claim them.
- Legality in all decisions through an explicit link with human rights legal standards in all processes and outcome measurements.

You can find out more details about the Charter at www.dementiarights.org, the Dementia Rights website.

In recent years, legislation in other parts of the UK has provided some support and rights for carers. There are two aspects to carers' legal rights: those that relate to carers and those that relate to the person for whom they are caring.

Carers' rights include:

- the right to have their own needs assessed by the local authority
- the right to receive direct payments so that they can choose what services to have
- rights in the workplace.

A carer's right to an assessment of need is set out in the Carers and Disabled Children Act 2000. This says that all carers aged 16 or above, who provide a 'regular and substantial amount of care' for someone aged 18 or over, have the right to an assessment of their needs as a carer from their local Social Services department. If there is more than one carer providing regular care in a household, both are entitled to an assessment.

The Carers (Equal Opportunities) Act 2005 ensures that carers have to be made aware of their right to an assessment. It also states that a carer's needs must be taken into account when undertaking an assessment. This means that if the carer wants to undertake training in order to return to employment, or wants to learn to drive, or has any training, education, employment or leisure-related needs, these can be met as a result of the assessment.

Direct payments are available to carers to support them to employ the services they need to assist them in their caring role. Many carers prefer to organise and employ support workers themselves, rather than have a service provided by the local authority.

Carers who are employed have the right to ask for flexible working if they live with the person they care for. Employers are not bound to grant these requests. However, they must give business reasons for refusing a request for flexible working. Carers also have the right to take unpaid time off work in an emergency relating to the person they care for.

The Equality Act 2010 gives carers the same protection from discrimination as the person they care for. This means that in matters such as buying goods and services – including shops, leisure facilities and access – the carer is also protected by the law against being treated any less favourably than someone who is not a carer.

4.3 Involving carers in planning support

The legal position in relation to people with dementia is that as long as they have capacity to make decisions, then they are in control of their own life. A carer can only act with the person's consent. However, if a Lasting Power of Attorney (LPA) has been put in place while the person still has capacity, then the carer can take the decisions identified in the LPA. If the person lacks capacity, and there is no LPA in place, the Court of Protection can appoint the carer as a deputy to enable them to take decisions in the person's best interests.

It is essential that all professionals work closely with family carers and that they are involved in all decisions regardless of the legal status. However, it is important to be clear that this can only be done with the consent of the person with dementia as long as they have capacity. It is not acceptable to discuss anything with a carer if the person does not agree.

Assuming that there is agreement from the person to the involvement of carers, then they should participate in all planning and review of support plans and packages. Alongside the person with dementia, carers should attend all meetings and reviews.

The principles of person-centred support planning mean that support should be planned in the following order:

1 What the person can do for themselves.
2 What family and informal carers are able to do.
3 What professional care support can do to fill the gaps.

4.4 How the need to protect may prevent rights and choices

It is not always easy for family carers to allow their loved ones to take risks. Very understandably, they want to protect them from harm.

Many carers can see the advantages of enabling people to make choices and take risks in order to improve their overall well-being, but some will find it difficult and will welcome support during the process.

4.5 Supporting carers to enable an individual to achieve their potential

Offering people examples of how people's lives have improved, and how much happier and more relaxed people are, can help. Sometimes it can be helpful to try a new approach for a short time in order to see how it works, and then gain agreement to continue if it is successful.

Where there are family and friend carers supporting a person with dementia, ongoing support and planning must always be a team approach, where everyone is involved. Family and friend carers should never be made to feel that they are less important than professional carers, and you must be careful not to take over their role.

Balancing rights and risks is the basis for this chapter, and this is just as important for carers. They need to be able to recognise the rights of their loved one, and the best way that they can be supported to balance the risks and reduce them as far as possible.

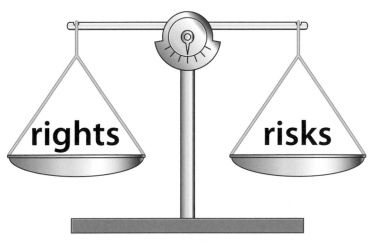

Figure 5.2: Balancing rights and risks is a huge challenge.

Getting ready for assessment

DEM 211 is all about balancing rights and risks. You will have to show that you understand why it is necessary for people to be able to take risks in order to exercise their rights to make choices about their lives. Your assessor will want to see that you have understood how risks can be used positively in order to support people to be in control and make choices about their lives.

This is a competence-based unit that assesses knowledge and demonstration of skills. You will need to demonstrate in a workplace setting that you are able to involve people and their carers and families in their own support. This means that you must show that people have chosen their support package as far as possible, and that families and friends have assisted with the process.

You need to have found out as much as possible about the person you are supporting and know how their history influences their present. Your assessor will want to see that you have used life history to help you to respond to people with dignity and respect.

Your assessor will also want to know what you do in your practice to make sure that people's rights are respected and that they are able to make choices and decisions about their lives.

Some of the assessment criteria ask for specific things. When you are asked to explain, do not simply list or describe. Use words such as 'because', 'as a result of', 'so that' and 'in order to'. If you are explaining something, you must show that you understand the reasons for it.

Glossary

Anti-discriminatory practice   working in ways that challenge discrimination.

Anxiety   feelings of nervousness, worry or unease.

Cerebral hemispheres   the key areas in the brain that are affected by the conditions and diseases that result in dementia; they make up most of the brain.

Delirium   mental confusion and changing levels of consciousness.

Dementia   a disability caused by diseases or conditions that affect the brain and that causes problems with the way the brain functions.

Depression   severe dejection, accompanied by feelings of hopelessness and being inadequate.

Diagnosis   identification of an illness by looking at the symptoms.

Discrimination   the result of behaviour that excludes, or fails to include, people.

Diversity   relates to difference and the richness and variety that different people bring to society.

Episodic memory   this holds information about events or 'episodes' in a person's life.

Equality   treating people equally: it is not the same thing as treating everyone the same.

Incidence   how many times something happens: always defined within a time frame (e.g. a year).

Inclusion   making sure that people are included and not left out.

Mental disorder   this term is used in the Mental Health Act 2007. Within the Act, dementia is considered to be a mental disorder.

Nearest relative   the person who looks after the interests of the person.

Personhood   all the essential things that make someone who they are – a status that recognises individuals in society.

Prevalence   how often something occurs.

Rementia   the improvement in dementia symptoms that can result from people being treated with respect and valued for the abilities they still have.

Risk assessment   identifying and evaluating risks.

Risk factors   the elements in someone's history or lifestyle that increase or decrease the chances of developing a particular condition.

Self-image (or **self-concept**)   how people see themselves.

Semantic memory   this holds information, facts and figures, and part of it stores words.

Stereotype   a generalised, oversimplified view of a particular type of person or thing.

Stereotyping   making assumptions that all people in a particular group are the same.

Stigma   a mark of disgrace associated with a particular circumstance, quality or person.

Stress   being under physical, mental or emotional pressure.

Symptoms   physical or mental indicators of a disease of injury.

Further reading and research

Websites

Alzheimer's Society

www.alzheimers.org.uk

The UK's leading care and research charity for individuals with dementia and those who care for them. The organisation provides information, support, guidance and referrals to other appropriate organisations. The website also has plenty of information on communicating with people who have dementia.

British Institute of Learning Disabilities

www.bild.org.uk

Works to improve the lives of individuals with disabilities. It provides a range of published and online information.

Careers Trust

www.carers.org

A new charity formed following the merger of The Princess Royal Trust for Carers and Crossroads Care. The website includes resources that focus on family carers for people who have dementia.

CJD Support

www.cjdsupport.net

An organisation which supports individuals with prion diseases, including forms of Creutzfeldt-Jakob disease (CJD). They provide a range of information on the various forms of prion disease, and work with professionals to improve the level of care provided for individuals with these conditions.

Dementia Positive

www.dementiapositive.co.uk

Useful resources on how to approach dementia in a positive and constructive way, as a result of the work of John Killick and Kate Allan.

Huntington's Disease Association

www.hda.org.uk

An association that provides information, advice, support and useful publications for families affected by Huntington's disease in England and Wales. It can put you in touch with a regional advisor and your nearest branch or support group.

Skills for Care

www.skillsforcare.org.uk

Works to support employers to ensure that care workers have the skills needed to provide high quality social care.

Social Care Institute for Excellence

www.scie.org.uk

In their Dementia Gateway section, there are a large number of resources that support working with people who have dementia, including case studies

Books

Lawrence, V., Samsi, K., Banerjee, S., Morgan, C. and Murray, J. (2010) 'Threat to valued elements of life: the experience of dementia across three ethnic groups', *Gerontologist*.

Milne A. and Chryssanthopoulou, C. (2005) 'Dementia care-giving in black and Asian populations: reviewing and refining the research agenda, *Journal of Community & Applied Social Psychology*, vol. 15, no. 5.

Townsend, J. and Godfrey, M. (2001) 'Asian experiences of care-giving for older relatives with dementia: an exploration of barriers to uptake of support services', Leeds: Nuffield Institute for Health.

Unit numbers by awarding organisation

Chapter no. in this book	Unit no. in this book	Unit Title	Unit accreditation no.	Edexcel unit no.	NCFE unit no.	CACHE/ OCR unit no.	C&G unit no.
1	DEM 201	Dementia Awareness	J/601/2874	13	14	DEM 201	4222–237
2	DEM 202	The Person-Centred Approach to the Care and Support of Individuals with Dementia	H/601/2879	14	15	DEM 202	4222–238
2	DEM 204	Understand and Implement a Person-Centred Approach to the Care and Support of Individuals with Dementia	F/601/3683	37	37	DEM 204	4222–239
3	DEM 205	Understand the Factors that can Influence Communication and Interaction with Individuals who have Dementia	T/601/9416	15	16	DEM 205	4222–240
3	DEM 210	Understand and Enable Interaction and Communication with Individuals with Dementia	A/601/9434	39	39	DEM 210	4222–243
4	DEM 207	Understand Equality, Diversity and Inclusion in Dementia Care	A/601/2886	16	17	DEM 207	4222–241
4	DEM 209	Equality, Diversity and Inclusion in Dementia Care Practice	Y/601/9277	38	38	DEM 209	4222–242
5	DEM 211	Approaches to Enable Rights and Choices for Individuals with Dementia whilst Minimising Risks	H/601/9282	40	40	DEM 211	4222–244

Knowledge units

Competence units

Index

Glossary terms are indicated by **bold** headings and page numbers.

A

active involvement 123–4
Adults with Incapacity (Scotland) Act 107
advocates 46, 75
age 23–4
    as risk factor for dementia 17–18
    younger people with dementia 93–5
alcohol as risk factor for dementia 19
alertness, changes in 16
Alzheimer's disease 12, 14–15
anti-discriminatory practice 89
anxieties of carers 125
anxiety 55
approved mental health practitioners 110
assessment of carers' needs 37
assessment preparation 25, 48, 76, 100, 128
assistive technology 23
attitudes
    about dementia 84–6
    of others 25, 124–5

B

behaviour changes
    as symptom 3
    younger people with dementia 95
behaviour of others 25, 124–5
beliefs about dementia 84–6
benefits for carers 38
best interests of individual with dementia 113–14
biographies 40–1, 54, 68–72, 78, 90–1, 118–19
black and minority ethnic (BME) community 96–7
body language 52–3, 63
brain
    cerebral hemispheres 4–5
    frontal lobe 4
    impact of dementia on 3–5
    parital lobe 4
    temporal lobe 4

C

capacity
    assessment of 106–7
    decision-making 111–12
care workers 46
carers
    anxieties of 125
    assessment of needs 37
    benefits and support for 38
    black and minority ethnic (BME) community 97
    communication with 36
    importance of 33
    information sharing with 35–6
    involvement in planning support 126–7
    involvement of 34–5
    potential of individual with dementia 127
    rights and choices of individual with dementia 127
    rights of 37, 125–6
    role of 33–4
    scenarios for 33–4
    support for 83–4
    understanding of dementia by 35–6
    vulnerable 39
    working with 36–40, 125–7
Carers and Disabled Children Act 2000 126
Carers (Equal Opportunities) Act 2005 126
causes of dementia
    Alzheimer's disease 12
    Creutzfeldt-Jakob disease 13
    fronto-temporal dementia 13
    HIV/AIDs 13
    Korsakoff's syndrome 13
    Lewy body dementia 13
    vascular dementia 12
cerebral hemispheres 4–5
codes of practice 111
communication
    adapting styles of 62–6
    anxiety 55
    with carers 36
    depression 55
    effects of dementia on 50–4
    environmental factors 56
    hearing impairment 64
    identity and uniqueness 66–8
    involvement of others 75–6
    life histories 54, 68–72
    and memory impairment 56–9
    mental health 55
    non-verbal 52–3, 63–4
    person-centred approach 59–68
    in person-centred approach 42–3
    physical conditions and pain 54–5
    pictures 63, 74
    positive person work 73–4
    problems 15

problems as symptom 3
strengths and abilities, recognising 59–61
techniques for positive interaction 72–4
verbal 51–2, 56–9, 62–3
visual impairment 64–5
written 52
community psychiatric nurses (CPN) 46
community support 22, 82–3, 125
conditions mistaken for dementia 6–8
consultant specialists 46, 47
Creutzfeldt-Jakob disease 13
criminal records checks 110–11
cultural attitudes 84

D
danger, lack of judgement concerning 15
decision-making 111–13
delirium as mistaken for dementia **6**–7
dementia
conditions mistaken for 6–8
defined **2**
symptoms of **2**–3
dementia care advisors 46, 47, 75
depression 6, 55
Deprivation of Liberty Safeguards (DoLS) 108–9
diagnosis 20
diet as risk factor for dementia 18
disabilities
learning 65–6
physical 65
disability, dementia as 11–12
discrimination 88–9
disorientation 14
diversity
defined **78**
ethnicity 96–7
importance of 78
needs and preferences 93–9
Down's syndrome, people with 98
dreams 16

E
early onset dementia 23–4
Eastern culture 84
eating habits 16
emotional space, respect for 117–18
environmental factors 11–12, 56, 120–5
episodic memory 57
equality 79–80
Equality Act 2010 103–5, 126
ethnicity 96–7

exercise as risk factor for dementia 18–19
experience of dementia. *see* living with dementia

F
family and friends, support from 21–2, 75, 124–5
family history as risk factor for dementia 19
friends, support from 21–2, 75
frontal lobe 4
fronto-temporal dementia 13, 16

G
gender as risk factor for dementia 18
genetics as risk factor for dementia 19
GPs 46, 75

H
hallucinations, visual 16
hearing impairment 54, 64
HIV/AIDs 13
human rights 102–3
Human Rights Act 1998 102–3

I
identity and uniqueness 66–8
impairment
hearing 54, 64
physical environment 120–3
visual 54, 64–5
see also memory impairment
incidence 19
inclusion 80–1
diverse needs 93–9
involvement of individuals in own care 92–3
life histories 90–1
valuing people 87–8
independence 123–4
independent mental capacity advocates (IMCA) 46, 47
independent mental capacity health advocates (IMCA) 110
independent mental health advocates (IMHA) 110
interaction. *see* communication

K
Kitwood's model 28–9
Korsakoff's syndrome 13

L
late-life forgetfulness compared to dementia 7–8
learning disabilities 65–6, 98–9
legislation 102–11, 125–6
Lewy body dementia 13, 15–16
life histories 40–1, 54, 68–72, 78, 90–1, 97, 118–19

lifestyle as risk factor for dementia 18–19
listening 64
living with dementia
    assistive technology 23
    attitudes and behaviour of others 25
    community support 22
    diagnosis 20
    early onset dementia 23–4
    professional support 22–3
    support from family and friends 21–2
    types of dementia 24
local communities 82–3, 125
long-term memory 57

M
medical model of dementia 8–9
medication, self-administration of 92–3
memory impairment
    and communication 56–9
    effects of 57, 59
    episodic memory 57
    functions of memory 56, 58
    long-term memory 57
    semantic memory 57
    sensory memory 56
    short-term 14
    as symptom 2
Mental Capacity Act 2005 105–7
mental disorder 109
mental health 55
Mental Health Act 2007 109–10
Mild Cognitive Impairment (MCI) compared to dementia
        7–8
misplacement of items 14
misunderstandings about dementia 84–6
mobility 15
models of dementia
    disability, dementia as 11–12
    medical 8–9
    social 9–11
mood changes 3, 15
movement problems 16

N
nearest relative 109
needs and preferences
    carers, support for 83–4
    diversity in 93–9
    and ethnicity 96–7
    importance of 82
    learning disabilities, people with 98–9

local communities 82–3
non-verbal communication 52–3, 63–4
nurses 46

O
occupational therapists 46
opportunities, taking 44–5

P
pain 54–5
parital lobe 4
person-centred approach
    adapting styles of communication 62–6
    applying 87–93
    benefits of 30–2
    and carers 33–40
    communication 42–3
    and communication 59–68
    involvement of individuals in own care 40–5, 92–3
    Kitwood's model 28–9
    learning disabilities, people with 99
    life histories 40–1
    needs and preferences 82–4
    opportunities, taking 44–5
    professionals, role of 46–8
    referrals 47–8
    risk identification and management 43–4
    strengths and abilities, recognising 59–61
    values underpinning 28
personal care, privacy for 115–16
personal space, respect for 117–18
personality
    changes in 16
    and life histories 40–1
personhood 59
pharmacists 46, 75
physical conditions and pain 54–5
physical disabilities 65
physical environment 120–3
physical space, respect for 116–17
physiotherapists 46, 47
pictures 63, 74
positive person work 73–4
preferences. *see* needs and preferences
prevalence rates **19**–20
privacy for personal care 115–16
professionals, role of 46–8, 110, 124
Protection of Freedoms Bill 2012 111
psychologists 46

R
reading 52
referrals 47–8
registration 111
rementia 28
responsible clinicians 110
rights of carers 37
rights of people with dementia
    achieving potential 120–5
    active involvement 123–4
    attitudes and behaviour of others 124–5
    best interests of individual with dementia 113–14
    codes of practice 111
    decision-making 111–13
    least restriction 114–15
    legislation 102–11
    life histories 118–19
    physical environment 120–3
    physical space, respect for 116–17
    policies and procedures 111
    privacy for personal care 115–16
    risk management 110–14
    social/emotional space, respect for 117–18
    social environment 123
risk(s)
    age 17–18
    alcohol 19
    assessments 43
    diet 18
    exercise 18–19
    family history 19
    gender 18
    genetics 19
    identification 43–4
    judgement concerning 15
    lifestyle 18–19
    management 43–4, 110–14
    smoking 18

S
self-image 66
self-medication 92–3
semantic memory 57
sensory memory 56
short-term memory 14, 56
signs of dementia. *see* symptoms of dementia
smoking as risk factor for dementia 18
social environment 123
social model of dementia 9–11
social space, respect for 117–18
social workers 46

speech and language therapists 46, 75
stereotypes 25, 88–9
stigma 85
stress as mistaken for dementia **6**
strokes 54
support
    achieving potential 120–5
    carer involvement in planning 126–7
    for carers 38, 83–4
    community 22
    and equality 80
    family and friends 21–2
    groups 46
    local communities 82–3
    professional 22–3
    for taking opportunities 45
symptoms of dementia **2**–3
    alertness, changes in 16
    Alzheimer's disease 14–15
    communication problems 15
    disorientation 14
    dreams 16
    eating habits 16
    fronto-temporal dementia 16
    Lewy body dementia 15–16
    misplacement of items 14
    mobility 15
    mood changes 15
    movement problems 16
    personality changes 16
    risk, lack of judgement concerning 15
    short-term memory loss 14
    slower thinking 15
    vascular dementia 15
    visual hallucinations 16

T
Talking Mats® 74
technology, assistive 23
temporal lobe 4
theoretical models of dementia
    disability, dementia as 11–12
    medical 8–9
    social 9–11
thinking, slower 15
touch 63

U
uniqueness 66–8

V

valuing people 87–8
vascular dementia 12, 15
verbal communication 51–2, 56–9, 62–3
visual hallucinations 16
visual impairment 54, 64–5
vulnerable carers 39

W

walking, problems with 15
Western culture 84
working relationship with carers 36–40
written communication 52

Y

younger people with dementia 23–4, 93–5

Z

zones of distance 118